ORGANIZED MEDICINE
IN THE PROGRESSIVE ERA

BY THE SAME AUTHOR

AMA: Voice of American Medicine

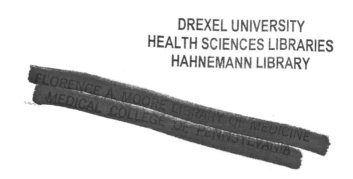
JAMES G. BURROW

Organized Medicine
in the Progressive Era

THE MOVE TOWARD
MONOPOLY

THE JOHNS HOPKINS UNIVERSITY PRESS

BALTIMORE AND LONDON

The Johns Hopkins University Press, Baltimore, Maryland 21218
The Johns Hopkins Press Ltd., London
Library of Congress Catalog Card Number 77–894
ISBN 0–8018–1918–0

Library of Congress Cataloging in Publication data will be found on the
last printed page of this book.

CONTENTS

PREFACE

This book grew out of compulsion to explore several areas in the economic and social history of the American medical profession that research on an earlier volume *(AMA: Voice of American Medicine)* suggested but did not allow. Long ago I became impressed by the way so many of the profession's policies and patterns of thought appeared to fall back on precedents set in the Progressive Era (1900 to 1917); the profession's principal achievements in this period seemed to lie at the state rather than at the national level. The research embodied in this volume has, in my opinion, confirmed these impressions and hopefully provides a clearer insight into the political behavior of the profession in recent decades. Despite frequent scholarly references to the political power of organized medicine, no extensive effort has been made to explain the process by which it secured this power at the crucial state level. Concentration on the advance and the limitations of state health and medical reforms, generally ignored by writers formulating theories of Progressivism, may provide better understanding of the period as a whole.

The outcome of the struggle over matters of health and medicine before the Progressive Era closed greatly affects all Americans as the last quarter of the twentieth century begins. Patterns of control that the profession secured over the supply of physicians in the Progressive Era account in large measure for the physician-shortage crisis that the nation has faced for about three decades. The public that has so recently witnessed the proliferation of doctoral diploma mills, grinding out disappointed unemployables in many fields, may find valuable lessons in the restrictive record of the medical profession in the Progressive Era. As the academic community watches the growth of menacing administrative bureaucracies in colleges and universities that terrorize faculties and threaten the instructional process, it may better understand the medical profession's attitude toward the "intermediate agent" who intervened between patient and doctor and demoralized the profession early in the twentieth century. And, too, as the nation struggles under the burden of medical bills that family budgets cannot bear and that voluntary plans often will not pay, it may appreciate some of the profession's ablest leaders of the Progressive period, who, deploring the rejection of a genuine social insurance plan, accurately predicted the plight that this generation would face in health and medical care.

The research for this volume rests substantially on the extensive published records of many state medical associations. These associations, listed in the Biographical Essay, comprised in their membership about two-thirds of the organized medical profession, and their publications reflect with reasonable accuracy the basic social and economic developments in the American medical world. Extensive research in the publications of most of the rival healing groups has helped to put the struggles of the medical profession in a broader setting. Several publications of the American Medical Association also added greatly to this study. Since indexes proved of little value in pointing the way to many of the obscure but significant developments within the profession in this era, many of the records of regular and irregular groups have been examined meticulously. Several private collections proved indispensable, and many monographs and government publications were of considerable help. But without the background work done on a related volume this book would not have been undertaken.

I am indebted to the personnel of some twenty libraries and depositories for assistance with this study. The staff of the National Library of Medicine allowed me ready access to many materials, and much of the research was conducted there. Useful material also was supplied by the staff of the Manuscripts Division of the Library of Congress. Eleanor Zinn of the Indiana University Medical School Library, and Eleanor Steinke, head librarian of the Library of the Vanderbilt Medical School, were very helpful. I should also like to acknowledge the assistance of Grace B. Horton, documents librarian, Library of the New York State School of Industrial and Labor Relations of Cornell University; Janet B. Koudelka, librarian of the Johns Hopkins Institute of the History of Medicine; Eleanor Wirmel, assistant librarian of the Museum of the Cincinnati Historical Society; and the staff of the Rockefeller Archive Center. At the Palmer School of Chiropractic, Davenport, Iowa, President David Palmer and Dean H. Ronald Frogley gave useful information, and at the Library of the Kirksville School of Osteopathy and Surgery, Kirksville, Missouri, Roberta Briscoe and Paula Nicholson were helpful.

Additional aid was provided through grants from the American Philosophical Society, Middle Tennessee State University, and Indiana State University. These financed a large part of the research.

I should like to acknowledge my indebtedness to Charles T. Gaisser of the History Department of North Alabama State University for many helpful suggestions, and to the late and eminent physician and writer, Max Seham of St. Paul, for sharing many ideas and offering much encouragement. I am especially indebted to Trudie Calvert, whose editorial criticisms and corrections of the manuscript were invaluable. Pat Shackelford of Abilene, Texas, was of much assistance in assuming most of the typing work. I am also indebted to Rhea M. and Barbara Burrow of Falls Church, Virginia, whose generous assistance lightened the burden of research in the Washington area. I owe the greatest debt to Robin, my wife, and to our children, Robin, Shannon, and Rachel who, to use the words of Robert C. Cook (*Human Fertility: The Modern Dilemma*), patiently tolerated my peevishness when I was "heavy with book." I alone assume full responsibility for any errors of fact or interpretation.

I A MEDICAL AWAKENING

CHAPTER ONE

M ERGING OF THE CENTURIES

Only hours before the chimes of Trinity, Grace, and St. Andrews Episcopal churches rang out the last moment of a dying year, the neighboring *New York Times* welcomed the approach of 1 January 1900, observed by many Americans as the beginning of a new century. Recounting some achievements of the nineteenth century that included revolutions in science and technology, the growth of democratic institutions, and seeming advance toward the peaceful settlement of international disputes, the *Times* editorial hoped that the new era would free mankind from the ancient scourges of war, poverty, and disease. It ignored the Boer conflict and the Philippine Insurrection then in progress as symbols of growing tensions and disorders, and, of course, it could not foresee the major reform movements that were about to appear on the American scene or the physical disasters, violence, and epidemics that soon would shake the nation.[1]

SPIRIT OF REFORM

Only scattered and sporadic protests of abuses in the social and economic order perpetuated dying agrarian agitation as the nineteenth century drew to a close. Reflecting lingering dissent, the *Arena* published in May 1898 the charges of Senator William M. Stewart of Nevada linking American finance capitalism with an international monetary conspiracy; a month later it carried an article in which John Clark Ridpath, writing on "The Invisible Empire," found a conspiracy against the public well established in the Senate. *Outlook* also introduced moderate protest of American materialism in 1899 by a Scottish author in "The Shadow on American Life." Spokesmen for reform organized the League of Social Service in 1898 and the National Conference on Social and Political Reforms a year later, but no indication of a sustained protest movement had appeared. Agitation remained uncertain and episodic as late as January 1900, when Arthur E. McEwen opened an attack in *Munsey's* on corporate graft.[2]

But protest literature increased within a year, and as dissenting groups became more outspoken the nation showed signs of moving into the major epoch of reform that later would be known as the Progressive Era. Caustic critics with a "passion for change" began to launch attacks on many fronts. By deriding some of the prominent crusaders as muckrakers, President Theodore Roosevelt provided a label that soon fell rather indiscriminately upon them all.[3]

Late in 1902 the muckraking era actually began when Claude W. Wetmore and Lincoln Steffens brought out in *McClure's* their first article exposing corruption in city government, followed by Ida M. Tarbell's serial account of the sordid practices of the Standard Oil Company. The novelist Frank Norris broadened the attack with an account of corruption among railroad and grain speculators, and the movement made perhaps its greatest impact when Upton Sinclair's *Jungle* portrayed the filth in the meatpacking industry just after Samuel Hopkins Adams had publicized medical quackery and patent medicine frauds. Federal food and drugs legislation followed in the wake of these exposures, and Norris's publicity, when added to the complaints of shippers and the desire of major railroads to reduce some forms of their competitive corruption, brought on significant federal controls.[4] But the mercurial muckraker, Thomas Lawson, saw no such results from his fierce indictment of crooked capitalism in "Frenzied Finance," nor did the upper house of the Fifty-ninth Congress suffer more than temporary shock from David Graham Phillips's attack entitled "Treason in the Senate." Yet the public had become more conscious of the power of corporate wealth as large industrial combinations sought ways to throw off the stigma of the trusts. Furthermore, Progressive leaders did not falter before corporate control or public inertia at the state level as they forced through reluctant legislatures important measures of social equity and political reform. They watched anxiously as federal courts retreated slowly from hallowed legal ground in accepting some restraints on the industrial oppression of working forces.[5]

VISITATIONS OF DISASTER

As the Progressive Era dawned, several tragic incidents drew greater public attention than did the sensational exposures later made by proponents of reform. Only eight months after the *New York Times* welcomed the year 1900, a fierce hurricane struck Galveston, Texas, and physicians gathering there for the annual meeting of the state medical association in April 1901 heard vivid accounts of the wreckage left in its path. James B. Stubbs, representing the mayor, welcomed the group as a part of the honored profession that faithfully had administered to the suffering city in its hour of tragedy, and prominent local physician Hamilton A. West described the horrors of that September night. Explaining that not all of the city's deaths were directly attributable to drowning, he added: "Some were crushed by falling timbers, some imprisoned beneath debris, some killed by flying slate, some knocked from floating rafts and either killed outright or so disabled as to be at the mercy of the raging waters."[6]

West described both the hurricane's destruction and the malarial epidemic that soon swept the city. Even though Alphonse Laveran had discovered the malarial parasite two decades before, Ronald Ross had identified the mosquito as the carrier in 1897, and Amigo Bignami and Giovanni B. Grassi the anopheles two years later, the Galveston physician thought that the disease also sprang from other sources. Finding no evidence of anophelene mosquitoes in the ruins and urging further etiological investigations, he expressed an uncertainty probably shared by a sizable part of the profession.[7]

As Galveston cleared away the debris and told the world of its losses, prominent political leaders in California moved to suppress the scientific report of a federal commission revealing conclusively that the dreaded scourge of the East, the bubonic plague, had reached San Francisco. The startled state medical association prepared for emergency measures as the death count in 1900 mounted rapidly following the first verified fatality on 6 March. Yet the mayor and California's governor seemed unconvinced and, in conflict with the medical association, remained as intractable as the disease itself. Obstructed by political forces but supported by scientific research that less than a decade before had discovered the bacillus of the plague and identified its carrier, the medical profession slowly brought the epidemic under control only to see it erupt again a few years later.[8]

Before the profession had succeeded in removing the anxieties of a troubled city, the presidential assassination of 6 September 1901 raised questions that struck at medical science on a more vulnerable front. Six physicians who examined William McKinley's assassin, Leon

F. Czolgosz, confirmed his sanity, and several were present at his execution in the Auburn penitentiary on 29 October, hearing the prisoner say calmly, "I killed the President because he was an enemy of the good people—the good working people. I am not sorry for my crime."[9] This estimate of the nation's leader one medical authority called "a false belief, but in no sense an insane delusion," and the autopsy in which the brain was removed and thoroughly examined showed no physical abnormalities. The observations of Edward A. Spitzka of the New York College of Physicians and Surgeons, who conducted the postmortem, revealed the uncertainties of a profession that had rejected some of the older theories of criminology but had traveled no great distance along more enlightened paths. "It is well known that some forms of psychosis have absolutely no ascertainable anatomic basis; and the assumption has been made that these psychoses depend rather upon circulatory and chemical disturbances. . . . Taking all in all, the verdict must be, 'socially diseased and perverted, but not mentally diseased.' The most horrible violations of human law cannot always be condoned by the plea of insanity. 'The wild beast slumbers in us all. It is not always necessary to invoke insanity to explain its awakening'."[10]

The new century so confidently greeted by most Americans had more shocks in store for those who thought that the nation's principal health problems lay largely in fighting disease in Spain's lost empire or in other areas beyond its own borders. Numerous reports of hookworm appeared in the last years of the nineteenth century, but in May 1902, a government scientist, Charles W. Stiles, identified and named a new species quickly detected as a major factor contributing to the erosion of human resources in the South.[11] Commencing a battle in which for years instances of infection multiplied far more rapidly than cures, the stricken region had little idea that its struggles would span several decades.

Long unable to stop the spread of hookworm, the South also fell prey to a more elusive menace that had emerged in Georgia in 1902. Pellagra had appeared, and as its victims multipled the bewildered medical profession fought frantically against a disease of unknown origin and uncertain cure.[12] By 1909, when pellagra cases had been discovered in thirteen states, and when total estimates of the affliction ranged from one thousand to five thousand, theories explaining its origin had spread more rapidly. Elaborate explanations attributed the disease to buffalo gnats, sand and stable flies, mosquitoes, clay soil, and even to residence in old mountain areas, but the theory gaining perhaps the earliest and widest acceptance traced its origin to spoiled corn. In the absence of convincing evidence accounting for the disease, however, the second triennial conference on pellagra in 1912 reported no certain cause or specific remedy, and nearly three years passed before its origin was traced definitely to dietary deficiencies.[13]

Other diseases spreading terror over the nation in the early twentieth century demonstrated all too frequently not only the limitations of scientific medicine but public inertia in appropriating its benefits as well. The use of mercury gave medical science some of its most impressive gains against syphilis, and physicians in the city of New York treated 162,372 cases of venereal infection in 1901 with it. A remedy, Salvarsan, often more effective, was discovered before the decade ended. A smallpox epidemic attacking Indiana in its most virulent form in December 1902 brought near panic to that state and the threat of suspension of trade by Kentucky, its most frightened neighbor, before adequate measures checked its advance. And while Indiana and later Ohio fought this scourge, a typhoid epidemic struck nearly 2,650 residents of Ithaca, New York, and later Butler, Pennsylvania, inflicting almost two hundred deaths.[14] In 1905, New Orleans, often the victim of pestilence, rallied its forces against another yellow fever attack. But the most deadly blow befell the city of New York two years later when infantile paralysis killed and maimed twenty-five hundred people in the most devastating attack ever reported in any part of the world. In the same year another threatening menace, soon to be known as tularemia, appeared unpublicized in the Arizona Territory and later struck with greater force in Tulare County, California, from which it derived its name.[15]

Besieged by diseases that often reached epidemic proportions, the nation also struggled against the stealthy attacks of the most dangerous perennial assailants. In 1900 cancer stood in eighth place among diseases causing death, accounting for considerably more fatalities than dreaded diphtheria that held tenth position. Yet the death rate for tuberculosis per hundred thousand of population more than tripled cancer casualties, while influenza and pneumonia surpassed even the white plague as the greatest destroyer of human life.[16]

ADVANCE IN SCIENTIFIC MEDICINE

Had physicians combated the diseases of the early twentieth century with no more than the near-empty arsenals of curative medicine their struggle would have been largely unavailing. Addressing the House of Delegates of the American Medical Association as late as 1903, President Frank Billings lamented that physicians had no specific remedies for most infectious diseases and that with the exception of quinine for malaria and mercury for syphilis drugs were "valueless as cures."[17] Fortunately, hopes for victory over disease did not altogether depend on the discouraging progress of curative medicine. In the field of preventive medicine the old century bequeathed to the new the momentum of several recent scientific triumphs.

Against diseases that long had concealed their origins, late nineteenth-century investigators made remarkable headway. Highlighting the accomplishments of the era were such achievements as the discovery of the pneumococcus, the malaria plasmodium, and the typhoid bacillus in 1880, and the bacillus of tuberculosis in 1882. The next year investigations isolated the diphtheria bacillus for which Emil von Behring developed an antitoxin in 1890. Before the end of the decade Anton Weichselbaum had isolated the meningococcus and Shibasaburo Kitasato had discovered the tetanus bacillus. Identification of bacilli causing influenza and the bubonic plague came early in the next decade and the discovery of the dysentery bacillus and filterable viruses before it closed.[18]

The new century, while portraying the limitations of scientific medicine with embarrassing frequency, brought forth spectacular achievements in preventive and curative medicine. In 1901 an American mission to Cuba produced conclusive proof that the mosquito, *stegomyia fasciata,* spread yellow fever. In 1905, Fritz Schaudinn isolated the bacillus of syphilis, and five years later Paul Ehrlich made successful use of his discovery, Salvarsan, in syphilitic treatments. Further investigations drawing on the research talents of several nations found the whooping cough virus in 1906, perfected a serum for meningitis in 1908, and discovered that the typhus was a lice-borne disease the next year.[19] The accomplishments of the era also included Karl Landsteiner's discovery of blood groups in 1901, the wider use of X-ray and radium, and bold and successful experimentation in lung, thyroid, prostatic, orthopedic, and neurosurgery. The work of Sigmund Freud, which attracted wide recognition just as the century began, opened up vast areas in the study of mental ailments, while James MacKenzie's heart research in London had gone far toward establishing cardiology as a major specialty by the end of the decade.[20]

The notable advance of world medicine in the second decade brought added American contributions although the gradual move of the United States toward World War I almost snuffed out the dimming light of political reform. Years of research bore fruit in 1911, when the first vitamin was discovered and in 1915 when Edward C. Kendall, an American physician, isolated the thyroid hormone. A year later a Japanese scientist demonstrated that skin cancer could be produced in animals by tar applications. The Great War itself provided a worldwide laboratory demonstrating the triumphs of scientific medicine, but near its close the great influenza epidemic sweeping much of the world and taking some twenty million lives dramatized in a ghastly way the limitations of medical advance.[21]

MEDICAL LEADERSHIP OLD AND NEW

When the achievements of the early years of the new century were blended with those of the last decades of the old, medical science had passed through its most triumphant era. Yet even a mere survey must depict the advance in more than scientific terms. Much of American medical progress in the old era and many of its hopes for the new were symbolized in 1900 by the overlapping careers of a notable group of aged physicians, others in the prime years of achievement, and still a younger group soon to achieve international renown.

Three eminent elderly physicians, all former presidents of the AMA, and all dying within a week of each other in September 1900, were Alfred Stillé, Lewis A. Sayre, and Hunter H. McGuire. Trained under the great French clinician, Pierre C. A. Louis, Stillé became a prominent medical educator and author and Sayre a renowned orthopedic surgeon and leader in New York's public health crusade. As a young medical instructor at Jefferson Medical College, McGuire first became widely known as the leader of three hundred southern medical students in their departure from Philadelphia for Richmond to protest Northern sympathy for John Brown's raid; he later became a prominent surgeon in Richmond. On 11 September death closed the career of another outstanding physician, Jacob M. Da Costa, whose textbook, *Medical Diagnosis,* passed through nine editions, remaining as a monument to his influence.[22] Within the next two years the profession lost

Christian Fenger, its most distinguished pathologist, and in 1904, Nathan S. Davis, "Father of the American Medical Association" and twice its president. Before the decade closed the death of Nicholas Senn, a famous Chicago surgeon, further detached the profession from the medical leadership of the old era.[23]

But as death cut quickly and deeply into the ranks of the nation's leading physicians, others of growing renown moved into the forefront. At the Johns Hopkins University School of Medicine the work of William Osler, Howard A. Kelly, William H. Welch, and William S. Halstead won international acclaim, and from Chicago the reputation of John B. Murphy, "the stormy petrel of surgery," rapidly spread abroad. The aging Abraham Jacobi continued to reign over the domain of pediatrics, and the noted surgeon, Christian Herter, worked on in the fame of his declining years. At an obscure Minnesota hamlet William J. Mayo and Charles H. Mayo built from small beginnings the famous Mayo Clinic, and before the Progressive Era closed the rural Kansas physician, Arthur E. Hertzler, had received wide recognition for his work in tumor surgery.[24]

An era that brought to American medicine growing international stature developed its talent for future leadership as well. The best of American medical schools offered outstanding training, and a few provided young specialists with unusual opportunities for teaching and research. On the widening ranges of medicine the peaks of personal genius became less imposing, but some promising specialists made outstanding contributions. Among these was George R. Minot, who, upon finishing Harvard Medical School in 1912, turned his attention to diseases of the blood, and along with another young physician, William P. Murphy, proved conclusively fourteen years later that pernicious anemia could be cured. The career of Harvey Cushing burst into full bloom at the end of the Progressive Era with the publication of *Tumors of the Nervus Acusticus* and with the growing success of his work in neurosurgery at Harvard.[25]

INTERNATIONAL CONTACTS

Although American medical progress in the Progressive Era began to free American medicine from Old World dominance, it also united as never before the scientific strivings of two continents. Major medical publications increasingly broadened their coverage of developments in international medicine, but contacts extended far beyond widening journalistic advance. The profession generally bestowed fitting tribute upon visiting international medical figures, and prominent American physicians gained great recognition abroad. Late in 1902, eager medical schools and clinics opened their doors to the great Viennese physician, Emil Lorenz, for demonstrations of his orthopedic treatments, while pitiful groups of the lame and crippled thronged in his path begging for cures.[26] Throughout the nation a saddened profession mourned in the same year the death of Rudolph Virchow, the world's most renowned pathologist, and six years later an appreciative medical group honored Robert Koch for his part in the struggle against tuberculosis, cholera, and sleeping sickness with a testimonial banquet in New York. On the panels of international medical assemblies leading American physicians took their places in growing numbers among established world figures, and at the International Surgical Congress in Budapest in 1909, the impression made by John B. Murphy was so favorable that three foreign participants yielded their time to extend his address.[27]

ROLE OF PHILANTHROPY

As American medicine moved toward a position of world leadership in the Progressive Era access to great reserves of private wealth assured its advance. From massive fortunes largely acquired in the scramble of the Gilded Age came contributions for medical institutions and research. Rockefeller philanthropy established the Rockefeller Institute for Medical Research in 1901, which began its work three years later, and in 1903, the General Education Board. In 1902, Andrew Carnegie established in the nation's capital the Carnegie Institute for the advancement of scientific research and subsidized the publication of the *Index Medicus* shortly after.[28]

Lavish outlays expanded select medical schools, stabilized some hospitals, and established others as philanthropists competed in disposing of their wealth. By 1902 the Harvard Medical School had received nearly $3 million in gifts from John D. Rockefeller, John Pierpont Morgan, and Mrs. Collis P. Huntington, and the New Maternity Hospital of New York City opening the same year owed its establishment to a $1 million Morgan gift. Later in the decade a sizable private grant established the Russell Sage Institute of Pathology as an adjunct of New York's City Hospital, but the era of lavish subsidization had only begun.[29]

A flush of philanthropy on the eve of World War I brought to the Cornell Medical School $4.35 million from an anonymous donor while the less modest Carnegie Foundation gave $1 million to the Vanderbilt Medical School. A $4.5 million gift from Peter Bent Brigham provided the Harvard Medical School with a new teaching hospital, erected in 1913, that bore his name. From the Rockefeller fortune went $1.5 million to the Johns Hopkins Medical School and $750,000 and $500,000 respectively to the medical institutions of Washington University and Yale in a thrust that raised its total gifts to medical education beyond $20 million by the end of the decade. A strenuous campaign to equip the University of Chicago with a medical school and a teaching hospital brought a sum from donors that reached $5 million as the Progressive Era closed.[30]

CHALLENGE AND ACHIEVEMENT

The union of wealth and talent in the struggle for better health in the new century gave rise to considerable hope. Yet even preventive medicine, which rapidly forged ahead, increasingly confronted barriers that yielded slowly, if at all, to scientific advance. Needless epidemics from sources that long before had been brought under scientific mastery showed clearly that much of the battle lay on political and social fronts. Forces promising to advance curative medicine had made only faltering moves.

Much within American medicine lay in disarray in 1900, but the Progressive Era established the foundations for a substantially different order. As voluntary lay protest groups rose to attack social and political abuses on many fronts, within the medical profession societies sprang up and others awakened from decades of dormancy to emphasize their own version of reform. A disheartened profession moved from virtual political impotence when the century began to a monopolistic control of medical practice before the era closed. Out of this period came a revolution in medical education that raised medical standards while widening opportunities for employing the techniques of guild control. During the era the foundation was laid for the regular profession's alliance with the law when it successfully used government power to achieve its goals.

The Progressive Era marked a crucial point in sectarian medical history when older, irregular bodies put up their last major drives to avert extinction and when newer sects survived the repressive efforts of the dominant profession but found their functions legally confined in very restricted roles. The conventional profession matched its success in curbing the activities of irregular groups with the employment of effective and lasting pressures within its own ranks for suppressing discord and dissent. During this era serious doubt arose within the profession about the adequacy of conventional methods for meeting the cost of medical care. For the last time in more than half a century there was effective professional support for replacing traditional patterns with a government program of compulsory health insurance.

CHAPTER TWO

THE GREAT DESIGN

The state of scientific medicine at the beginning of the twentieth century caused recurring moods of confidence and frustration within the profession. There was little reason for confidence at the level of actual practice. Few physicians could practice by the best standards of the era, and the public promoted mediocrity in medicine by its own apathy and by its failure to expect better. Economic necessity often combined with casual scientific knowledge to turn physicians toward supplementary sources of income as competition, inflation, advance of preventive medicine, and the popularity of self-medication diminished their chances of economic survival. Arthur E. Hertzler cited no unusual instance when he referred to a neighboring Kansas physician, who, near the end of the nineteenth century, so closely combined hog raising with medical practice that he did not allow even a simple hand-washing ritual to separate the former occupation from the latter.[1]

STATUS REVOLUTION

The concept of "status revolution" serves partially to account for the volume of reform energies that swelled up in the ranks of medicine early in the Progressive Era. This concept, employed by Richard Hofstadter to explain the role of a displaced elite in the vanguard of political reform movements, has an application in the medical world that apparently he did not observe.[2] Physicians dwelling in modest comfort throughout most of the nineteenth century suffered from the inflation that began before it closed. No secular theme recurs more frequently in the medical literature of the Progressive Era than that of the hardships imposed by inflation and static or falling incomes. Nor did physicians feel that all other groups shared their distress. With only partial accuracy one prominent journal expressed in 1910 what many others had observed: "There are perhaps none in the community, with the possible exception of the small salaried men, who suffer more . . . than do physicians. The wage earner has seen his wages steadily increase with the increased cost of living; the storekeeper makes the same margin of profit, or a larger one, than before; . . . but the medical man . . . sees his income steadily diminish . . . and his dollars shrink in size."[3]

THREATENING POVERTY

Ample income statistics strengthened physicians' fears of the approach of widespread professional poverty. A study conducted in 1902 showed that more than 100,000 of the approximately 135,000 physicians in the United States made less than $1,500 a year, while another in 1907 reported that most country doctors made no more than $1,200.[4] A survey of nine states in 1907 indicated no rise whatever in physicians' incomes in twenty-five years despite an increase in the cost of living of about 24 percent in only one decade. A report of the income of physicians in seventy-nine Texas counties the same year showed an average income of $1,873, but that 1,709 out of 3,317 physicians (52 percent) barely made a living.[5]

Alert physicians easily discovered the cause of their plight. The number of institutions purporting to offer medical training rose from 90 in 1880 to 154 in 1903. A total of 27,615 students poured into these schools for the session that closed in the latter year and 5,698 graduates poured out, bringing panic to the profession and dismay to its leadership. Not only did medical schools flood the field, but the saturation occurred largely at the lowest levels of competence. For every graduate who entered the profession from a reputable and established school, a score of others found ready entrance through transient proprietary enterprises. When even the best of institutions confessed to the limitations of their academic programs, proprietary establishments had to capitalize on their ease and leniency as reasons to exist.[6]

Frightening competition and the degraded standards of medical schools illustrated the near futility of the American Medical Association's half-century struggle for educational reform. But the situation pointed up the public's incapacity to deal with the growing crisis, as legislatures made scant effort to control entrance into the profession by adequate licensing statutes.[7] To leaders of American medicine the spectacle of political and professional impotence suggested something more: only a professional and political alliance, they concluded, would bring about reform.

TURN TO POLITICS

The demonstrated political impotence of organized medicine, the growing threats to scientific medical advance, and the darkening economic outlook shook the American profession as no other set of developments ever had. These provocations brought forth a leadership that could clarify and express the profession's grievances. This leadership transformed the spreading ferment of unrest into nationwide agitation that brought the profession from political obscurity to public prominence in less than one decade. It gave the AMA mastery of the techniques of mass appeal; enormous political leverage, state and national; and consummate skill in mingling public interest with its own.

No event in the social history of American medicine is more important than the selection in 1900 of the magnetic secretary of the Kentucky State Board of Health to organize the medical profession. The prominent physician William W. Keen of Philadelphia, chairman of the AMA's Committee on Reorganization, saw in the personable Kentuckian, Joseph N. McCormack, qualities of leadership that he thought could unite the scattered remnants of organized medicine into an effective force for political reform, and he persuaded McCormack to accept the work. As official organizer of the AMA, McCormack commenced a two-year program of visiting officials of state organizations and then an exhaustive campaign, lasting for nearly a decade, among city, county, and district societies of every state.[8]

McCormack was a leader who had overcome countless hardships to become a seasoned veteran of many political struggles to improve health in his native state. He was born near Bardstown in 1847, the sixth of sixteen children; his lineage included some families of local prominence and a maternal grandmother who was a close cousin of Andrew Jackson. Deprived of formal public education at the age of thirteen, he struggled alone to extend his learning and entered the Medical Department of the Miami University of Cincinnati in 1868. When he graduated as valedictorian, his concern for controversial social issues appeared in his class address on the mental and physical equality of the sexes. Although his outstanding surgical skills soon brought conferral of the ad eundem M.D. degree by the University of

Louisville, McCormack sought further study in 1882 with six months of postgraduate work in Europe.[9]

Shocked by the ravages of epidemics that swept his state and stricken along with other members of his father's family with typhoid fever in 1872, he decided to devote much of his time to the political demands of public health. In 1880 he was appointed to the state board of health and became its secretary two years later. He wrote all of Kentucky's public health measures and frequently fought strong opposition to secure their passage. He drove through the legislature the state's first medical practice law in 1888, bringing, for the first time in any state, representatives of the eclectic, homeopathic, and regular groups together to administer the act. He waged a relentless battle against professional quackery and in 1898 successfully led in the struggle to reorganize and revive the state's feeble medical association. When he brought the same dynamic spirit to the position of national organizer of the AMA, few could question that the reorganization committee had chosen wisely.[10]

THE ALABAMA IDEAL

With the inauguration of its expansion program the AMA broke a half-century precedent by subordinating its principal objective of advancing scientific medicine to the achievement of political goals. Nearly two decades of struggle in Kentucky's public health battles had convinced McCormack that only political pressure from organized medicine could protect the public's health and the profession's interest. In the lower South the work of Jerome Cochran in transforming the Alabama profession into a strong political force long had inspired the AMA. Contending that "the primary and principal object" of the Alabama association was not "the cultivation of the science and art of medicine" but the establishment of the society as a *medical legislature* having for its highest function the governmental direction of the medical profession of the state," Cochran found in Alabama's Reconstruction rubble a prostrate profession and from it created the most powerful association in the nation in less than a decade.[11] His five objectives were to unify physicians in Alabama, to improve their competence by frequent meetings devoted partially to scientific matters, to establish high standards for medical practice, to construct an adequate public health program, and to provide professional courts that would exercise jurisdiction over matters of ethics. As the AMA well knew, the Alabama profession had elected a majority of physicians to both houses of the state legislature in 1873, written the medical practice act four years later, secured passage of effective health legislation in the 1880s, and made each county society an integral part of the state government. Through Cochran's efforts state and local societies had become the state and local boards of health with authority over public health problems and control over admission into the profession.[12]

As the leadership of the AMA devised its strategy for organizational expansion it drew confidence and hope from the example of the Alabama society. At the annual session of 1901, President Charles A. L. Reed spoke of the "incomparable" Alabama association, and a year later, George H. Simmons, secretary of the AMA and editor of its *Journal,* observed the society when visiting the state and called it the best in the world and its structure and functions suitable for duplication in all but perhaps two mountain states. In his organizational crusade McCormack never tired of recounting the profession's struggles there or of citing the lasting effectiveness of Cochran's work.[13]

THE ANVIL CHORUS

Hoping to match Cockran's achievements in every state, McCormack brought to his work an organizational talent matching the difficulty of his task. As a medical evangelist with the nation as his parish, his highest priority was to promote unity within a discordant profession. Though long aware that hatreds divided physicians of his native state, he found as he moved over the nation that "from the lakes to the Gulf and from the Atlantic to the Pacific this black cloud of envy and jealousy hung over the profession."[14] Charging that such a professional spirit restricted itself to no particular age or culture, he cited Fra Albertus of the Middle Ages who wrote: "And the sons of Aesculapius, every mother's son of them took two or three hammers in his kipsey beside the one he had constantly in use on his brethren, and the only song they ever sang was the anvil chorus."[15]

McCormack believed that the wreckage wrought by this spirit lay everywhere. Physicians consumed time useful for the development of their professional talents in degrading personal strife. They quarreled, he said, about "diagnoses in which probably both were wrong; about patients who would not pay either of them, or about violations of the code, which neither of them had ever read."[16] Even families of feuding doctors bore the strain as rival wives warred with or avoided each other. McCormack charged that such exhibitions only tarnished the profession's image and brought no participant any gain. The public, he thought, readily accepted what doctors said about each other. Furthermore, he contended that "behind every malpractice suit there skulks some back-biting, envious doctor," seeking to destroy the resources and reputation of another.[17]

Nor did the injuries inflicted by dissension fall wholly on the profession. The Kentucky health official often saw professional hatreds overcome the urgencies of a local crisis and retard the adoption of emergency health measures. Disaffected physicians, he insisted, would rather call an approaching smallpox epidemic a visitation of elephant itch than concur in the decision of others. Not surprisingly, so divided a profession carried little or no political weight. McCormack found that legislators seldom trusted doctors and that professional endorsement of a measure often was tantamount to defeat.[18]

MC CORMACK'S APPEAL FOR UNITY

McCormack thought he found causes and cures for the dissensions that beset the profession. All largely unorganized vocations composed of individuals who rendered their services in isolation generated disruptive frictions. Among bankers, he insisted, enormous strife prevailed, and among the clergy only the growing success of local fellowship meetings had dissolved perennial discords. Lawyers, thrown together frequently, and often in court conflict, generally arose above professional bickering. McCormack charged that they would not argue at all unless paid in advance. Doctors, though, nursed their injuries, whether custom-made or home-manufactured, and allowed no statute of limitation to apply against them.[19]

Yet the segregated lives of physicians only partially accounted for professional discord. McCormack traced much of the friction to the bitter rivalry between medical schools and to their diffusion of this spirit among their graduates. He believed the professional strife that made his organizational efforts so difficult in Louisville and Dallas grew out of the bitterness aroused by local medical schools. Nor was he surprised to find that medical institutions offering little else provided the most generous quantities of this spirit.[20]

Of the assortment of causes contributing to professional frictions, McCormack never doubted that economic and social rivalry outweighed all others. Several years after his organizational campaign ended, he expressed a long-held view that difficulties "large and small, in city and country, are directly traceable to rivalry and jealousy between local doctors who are in each other's way or think they are." McCormack also recognized that the inflation of the first decade had only increased jealousy in a profession in which real incomes so often had diminished steadily.[21]

McCormack offered urgent proposals for reducing professional friction. He called for rigid adherence to an ethic requiring that no physician ever speak disparagingly of another. He urged every doctor to take a vow that "so long as God shall let me live, I will never say an unkind word of a fellow doctor." Employing biblical terminology to describe the abuse physicians inflicted verbally, he called the mistreatment of young physicians "an unpardonable sin," and only "a little milder sin to mistreat an old one."[22]

MC CORMACK ORGANIZES THE PROFESSION

McCormack's proposal for reducing dissension among physicians appeared to be no match for the malady. Yet he made the appeal for unity a part of a larger drive to organize vigorous medical societies over the nation. Attributing strife in a large measure to the segregated order of professional practice, he hoped to counter the divisive effects of this order through organization. Physicians, he claimed, not only would see strife diminish with the creation and invigoration of medical societies, but these societies would give them political stature and national influence. Not surprisingly, then, an organizational drive of national proportions ranked with the promotion of unity as one of McCormack's major goals.

The crusade that carried McCormack throughout the nation into most of the counties of every state and into perhaps more than two thousand towns and cities may well rate as the most fateful undertaking in the AMA's history. Pressing state societies to accept a cohesive organizational plan, which the AMA only recently had adopted, McCormack found most state associations cordial and compliant. But as he quickly learned, the creation of new societies and the infusion of purpose and life into many more that were aimless and inactive made overwhelming demands on his energy and talent. Speaking to groups of physicians as often as four times daily, and occasionally more, he felt first the warmness of their welcome and then the chilling effect of apathy and dissension that their best efforts could scarcely conceal.[23]

Undismayed by indifference and division, McCormack set before physicians everywhere the importance of his mission. His charismatic qualities usually aroused stirrings of revival in societies dead for decades. But personal magnetism alone did not account for his success in bringing on an awakening. Much power lay in the strength of his message voicing the complaints of a depressed profession, calling for a reaffirmation of its highest principles, and announcing the approach of a brighter era. Striking at the roots of rivalry, he denounced unethical advertising, secret fee splitting, abuses of contract practice, and medical quackery. He called for the strengthening of medical education and for the inclusion in the curriculum of a course in medical ethics, announcing that he would warn all prospective medical students to avoid any school that offered no such instruction. Proclaiming a surplus only of incompetent physicians, he declared that "if every patient were treated scientifically, there are not doctors enough in America to treat them all."[24]

Just as fearlessly, McCormack denounced the evils that threatened the profession from without. He deplored public apathy on matters of public health and the failure of politicians to follow the enlightened guidance of physicians in areas only they could understand. Repeatedly, he condemned the patent medicine interests as a prosperous enterprise based on deception and extortion. Nor did he forget the encroachments of druggists, with their prescription substitution and counter doctoring, on medical practice. Deploring the poverty of physicians and the lack of public concern for their welfare, he encouraged the adoption of moderate fee schedules to curtail the effects of ruinous competition.[25]

All too often McCormack found that societies caught up in the enthusiasm of his crusade fell back into indifference and that some he organized did not become active. Councilors in state societies frequently complained that they could not sustain interest in their districts. At least two state societies appointed organizers, and occasionally the AMA sent solicitors from its Chicago headquarters to recruit members. But before the middle of the decade McCormack found a more effective means of building and sustaining local memberships. He urged societies to offer physicians postgraduate courses of instruction on medical subjects closely related to their practice. Under his direction the AMA prepared schedules to assist societies in starting their programs.[26]

In 1909 over two hundred local organizations had responded to his appeal and many expressed growing interest in the program. McCormack proudly cited cases of unusual accomplishment, not ignoring rural areas where obstructions to real achievement seemed most forbidding. He reported the success of his work in a remote Kentucky county where four estranged physicians had agreed to forget their difficulties and pool their talents. Upon his suggestion three of them had taken postgraduate courses at major medical centers in preparation for more specialized practice on their return.[27] But McCormack asked most societies only to inaugurate locally directed postgraduate courses. He told physicians in twenty-two Michigan audiences that all Michigan doctors could have access to any information available to doctors of New York and Berlin and that he hoped to bring every family in the nation within reach of a competent, modern physician through his postgraduate program.[28]

The county society, rather than district or state organizations, ever remained McCormack's chief concern as he called for nothing less than a grassroots revival. "I believe the thorough organization of the profession is possible," he said, "only through the organization of county societies," arguing further that the "evils from which we are suffering are entirely local." Just as many reformers of the Progressive Era called for a quickening of political interest among the electorate, so McCormack attempted to arouse concern among what he called the "submerged two-thirds" who had lost scientific and professional contacts and political influence.[29]

MC CORMACK APPEALS TO THE PUBLIC

Despite the success that accompanied McCormack's work of building medical societies and promoting professional unity, he gradually recognized the inadequacy of his efforts. Convinced that the profession must establish a favorable public image, he added the cultivation of better public relations as a third crusade objective. Though laymen had appeared in many of his early audiences, not until after he had spoken at the San Antonio session of the Texas medical association in 1903 did he resolve to appeal to the public as part of his work. Speaking in this southern city to judges, lawyers, legislators, and other laymen, at a session in which he exposed the inadequacy of public health laws and the extent and evils of quackery and the patent medicine menace, he found that "only the plain common-sense instruction which fearless, progressive physicians alone can give was needed to enlist their active interest."[30]

McCormack encountered no difficulty in appealing to the public with arguments that identified the profession's interest with its own. In 1906 he wrote, "It has been found easy to demonstrate to any intelligent layman that his physician, and the profession as a whole, . . . [have] no interest which he does not share and that the daily safety and well-being of his family . . . [are] inseparable from the continued prosperity and competency of his physician and of the profession of his county, State and country as a whole."[31] In a pamphlet entitled "Dr. McCormack's Advance Agent," which announced plans for his organizational work within a state, McCormack sought to attract the interest of the public and the profession alike. This pamphlet emphasized that he offered no "dry, technical, scientific lectures" and that he had no addresses designed for physicians only. Furthermore, it stated that he would seek to remove public prejudice against physicians and to inform laymen of the public dangers that lurked behind the spectacle of an impoverished profession.[32]

The titles of McCormack's addresses suggest much of their appeal. Frequently he spoke on "Things about Doctors Which Doctors and Other People Ought to Know." He received wide acclaim for another address called "The Danger to the Public from an Unorganized and Underpaid Medical Profession." Another address he entitled the "Interrelations of the Profession and the People." Toward the end of the decade many audiences heard his lecture on "The New Gospel of Health and Long Life." By this time McCormack had set a public relations record for distance traveled and public audiences addressed that almost certainly no contemporary spokesman for any business enterprise or any other professional organization even remotely matched.[33]

McCormack's charm and magnetism showed up on the public platform, and the favorable image he projected served the profession as a whole. He allowed no affected modesty to conceal his familiarity with the profession as he spoke to audiences of his arduous schedule and suggested that he knew more American physicians than did any other five hundred men.[34] With such a knowledge of the profession he disarmed captious laymen with a frank recital of its sins. He found the nation crowded with inadequately trained physicians who had forgotten a large part of what little they had learned. Professional faults and abuses that local physicians often either denied or only privately acknowledged he now publicly confessed. Some, he acknowledged, had succumbed to the economic pressures of the era and had tarnished the profession's image by recourse to fee splitting, advertising, and yielding to the abuses of contract practice schemes.[35]

McCormack followed a vicarious confession of the profession's faults with a reaffirmation of its ideals. Ethical standards, placed by the profession on itself through centuries of struggle, far exceeded public demands. No physician could patent, conceal, or profit from a medical invention of his making. Willingly doctors had supported measures of public health that held out for them the prospect of declining incomes.[36] Moreover, the enormous charity work of the profession demonstrated substantial commitment to high ideals. Many doctors in the large cities, he observed, walked through hospitals two hours daily administering to the poor, while "country doctors, the noblest specimens of God's manhood, when called through the rain or shine, night or day, treat the rich and poor alike." He named several of the nation's leading physicians who gave much of their time to "tramps and hobos, to God's poor, the devil's poor and the poor devils." Without minimizing the benevolent work of churches, he said that physicians "gave more in charity than all the churches, benevolent orders, Christian Endeavors and Epworth Leagues combined." He cited a study that he and others had made of the charity work of the profession in Kentucky in 1904, which showed that at normal charges it reached a sum exceeding the total annual state, county, and city revenues and that one-half of the people in the state never paid their medical bills.[37]

Having made a disarming and assuasive appeal, he moved on to areas where public and professional interests quite obviously converged. Laymen in his Michigan audiences heard that one-half of the deaths in the state in 1905 came from preventable diseases. Proper preventive measures, he said, could stop the spread of tuberculosis that afflicted some twenty-five thousand residents of the state. He branded typhoid as an easily preventable filth disease and showed that diphtheria, scarlet fever, and cholera infantum could be controlled. Nor did he overlook the prevalence of venereal infections. He charged that "half of the diseases contracted through the immorality of young men are treated by little boy clerks in drug stores." Then he added that these men, mistakenly confident of cures, go out to marry your sisters and daughters, spreading a type of infection that accounted for one-half of all the surgery performed on women annually. Could not physicians and laymen join in destroying the nostrum industry that helped to spread contagious diseases and that passed off as a cure cheap whiskey that bore an exorbitant price when labeled as a patent medicine? He contended that state health departments and a proposed national department, if adequately equipped to inform the public of health hazards and to prevent the spread of disease, would have a value to the public as great as its judicial system.[38]

CALL FOR A COALITION

McCormack knew that the profession had alienated potential allies. He sought not only unity among physicians but their alignment with laymen in a movement to protect the nation's priceless asset, the public's health. Touching on sources of community leadership, he urged doctors to seek the support of lawyers and public officials. Aware that women had become more active in public affairs, he urged that physicians also enlist their aid. He appealed to teachers to educate the nation's youth on health and medical issues. McCormack called upon physicians and druggists to resolve their differences and to pursue their common goals. He proposed the creation of a coalition led by physicians that would make legislative bodies for the first time generally responsive to their demands. No longer need the divided forces of the profession retreat before the compact legions of quackery. He insisted that local societies and family physicians explain the principles of health and medical legislation to prospective legislators while they were still candidates, claiming that "nearly every vote can be controlled by education, moral suasion, and home influence in advance."[39]

Emphasis on the triadic goals of McCormack's program does not adequately portray the difficulty and complexity of his task. Fifty-three years of age when his crusade started and nearing old age when it closed, McCormack maintained a schedule that would have exhausted many younger and lesser men. In 1906 he addressed fifty assemblies in Illinois in twenty-five days and some forty more in Alabama during a similar period near the end of the year and just beyond, speaking to the Alabama legislature as well. In his second organizational effort in Ohio in 1908, lasting less than four weeks, he spoke in twenty-four cities in a campaign demanding no greater endurance than many of his others.[40]

The enthusiasm that McCormack generally aroused provided personal inspiration for his mission. Following his organizational work in Illinois, the council of the state medical association reported that if he could have stayed another month every possible engagement date would have been filled. State newspapers carried prompt and favorable comments on his Ohio campaign, and the organization of several public health leagues followed his work. An Akron audience of fifteen hundred packed a church auditorium to hear one of the last addresses of his statewide crusade, and many were turned away.[41] The Board of Censors of the Alabama association praised his work among physicians and laymen of the state, adding that "the address to the joint houses of the legislature helped very materially to place that body in a friendly attitude toward legislation desired by the organized medical profession."[42]

Not every greeting accorded McCormack was one of welcome nor every report of his visits one of praise. Professional audiences did not always respond favorably to his appeal, and not every statewide canvass came to a successful close. Noting his apparent failure to inspire Kansas physicians with the idealism of his crusade, McCormack spoke of their "almost universal and absolute indifference to every professional interest which was not strictly and immediately personal."[43] Confronting an apathetic profession unprepared for his first organizational work in Ohio in 1906, he stopped his tour abruptly and left the state. After he exposed factionalism among physicians of Oregon following his visit there in 1905, leading physicians of Portland protested that they deserved no such attack. McCormack's work in Illinois brought on a conflict with the state board of health and further opposition from an implacable enemy, G. Frank Lydston, a prominent Chicago medical professor.[44] Not surprisingly, leaders of sectarian medical movements opposed his work. His appearance in Kirksville, Missouri, brought an attack from officials of the local osteopathic school who correctly saw in McCormack's crusade a threat to their system. Patent medicine interests denounced McCormack because he had effectively exposed their trade as a public menace.[45]

MC CORMACK'S WORK EVALUATED

No single standard can serve to evaluate McCormack's special promotional work for the AMA which he terminated in December 1911. But by almost any test there passed from the limelight the most influential political leader of the profession in the Progressive Era, or perhaps, in the AMA's entire history. While other leaders of the AMA worked for measures affecting medical practice and public health at the federal level, he confined his activities largely to the states, in whose legislatures the greatest battles for the profession were fought and often won. While others dreamed of mobilizing the political energies of medicine over the nation through what was all too often a labyrinth of committees functioning only on a paper pad, McCormack sought through personal contact to imbue the system with spirit and life.

Perhaps the highest estimate of McCormack's work came as a tacit acknowledgement from the AMA itself only a year before it declined to choose him over another distinguished nominee for the presidency, its greatest honor. In 1910, when the AMA reorganized its promotional and publicity work, it accepted much of the program that McCormack had perfected in the first decade, but it devised a more complicated system of meeting the problem of public relations and expansion. In the new Council on Health and Public Instruction it established several bureaus, including one on medical legislation, another on public relations, and a third on organization. Appropriately, it called upon McCormack to head the latter, and, with other directors, he launched the broader program. Through the Bureau of Public Relations the AMA made materials on public health available to thousands of newspapers and journals and through a Speaker's Bureau and a Bureau of Literature, created only a short time later, it perpetuated much of McCormack's original program.[46]

An evaluation of McCormack's service requires more than simple acceptance of the profession's estimate of its worth. Although many physicians found him ideally suited for his task, few seemed to recognize that the AMA had brought to the front probably the greatest master of public relations the nation had yet produced. Nor is it clear that tempered modern judgment should assign to him a much lesser rank. Certainly he set a record in the twentieth century before World War I that no widely acclaimed public relations expert can even remotely match.[47]

The organization he so greatly strengthened reflects the enduring quality of his work. McCormack knew that some societies caught in the updraft of his promotional effort would lose much of their original fervor and that a few would not survive. But he believed correctly that a great number established or revived by his crusade would carry his work forward.

McCormack stood before the profession primarily as an advocate of organization, but he appeared before the public in a somewhat different role. He projected the image of the new physician, one trained by advancing scientific standards, sensitive to social issues, and culturally mature.[48] Much more than he ever realized, he had established for the profession what usually became contradictory goals. The growing demands of medical science not only tended to isolate physicians from each other in areas of specialization but also blocked the inflow of ideas from other professional fields. Increasingly, as physicians viewed the outer world largely through the constricted openings of private practice, they failed to grasp the complexity of the social burdens that an advanced technology had imposed. Insofar as they accepted the idea of scientific self-sufficiency, an acquaintance with their cultural heritage seemed to them increasingly irrelevant and remote. McCormack tried to bring to the new order much of value within the old and met substantial defeat before impersonal forces that he only vaguely understood and could not appreciably control.

II FERMENT AND REFORM

CHAPTER THREE

REFORM OF MEDICAL EDUCATION

Not even McCormack's organizational crusade of the early twentieth century could bring order to a profession that had become all but unmanageable. The rivalry between medical systems bred jealousy and detachment, and strife among physicians within regular and irregular healing groups only increased professional friction. Hordes of ill-trained doctors who could no more raise the scientific standards of the profession than the level of its ethics annually joined the ranks of medicine. Nothing less than a thorough reform of medical education for which the American Medical Association had struggled futilely for over half a century could check the ruin that faced the profession.

THE DEGRADED PROFESSION

Leading medical educators and editors of the early twentieth century deplored the low standards of medical education and the general quality of its products. At the Tulane University School of Medicine, George Dock testified to the virtual illiteracy of his third-year students whose assaults on orthography included "inflaimed," "bowalls," "simptom," "tetnas," "puss," and "irruption." Lincoln Cothran, as a member of the California State Board of Medical Examiners, found graduates in their "untutored earnestness" offering such approximations as "tung," "bludvescles," "dyafram," "uren," and "recktum." Henry Beates, Jr., president of the Medical Council of Pennsylvania, declared that of the papers he graded on licensing examinations some 30 or 40 percent represented appalling examples of illiteracy. George M. Gould, a prominent medical editor, complained that three-fourths of the four thousand annual graduates of medical institutions could not practice medicine intelligently.[1] Laying much of the blame for degraded stand-

ards on commercial medical colleges, Charles H. Wallace, while president of the Missouri Medical Association observed, "These student
hunters entice the barber from his chair, the mechanic from his bench
and the huckster from his wagon, all with imperfect education, and
push them by roseate pictures into the field of medicine. What can
such conditions bring forth [he asked] but imperfectly-feathered
fledglings who flutter along the marshes and never rise to the dignified
heights of the real physician [?]"[2]

From the hinterland came convincing evidence that physicians did
not often overcome the deficiencies of their education through medical
practice. A Georgia practitioner and graduate of a "reputable" medical
school inquired of a colleague if he had "airy" instrument to deal
with a patient whom he had found in a "catamose" condition. An
Arkansas physician, signing his letter "yours in nede," wrote of a
"pashunt whose phisical sines shose that the windpipe hav ulcerated
off and his lungs have dropped into his stumick." As late as 1901, residents of Quincy, Illinois, could employ the services of one practitioner
who found a patient in serious "trobel with his hart and brane" and
with blood in a "terabel cheaflus condition."[3] While physicians with
these limitations did not represent the profession's level of academic
attainment, they constituted a class that appeared with alarming frequency in all sections of the nation.

GOALS OF THE AMA

Well aware of the deficiencies in medical education, the AMA with
its affiliated societies began and largely completed a drive for fundamental reforms in the Progressive Era. Its demands for sweeping
reforms in the educational structure left no area of medical education
untouched. In attempting to reduce competition in the profession and
to elevate its standards it sought to control the entrance requirements
of medical schools. For the same purposes it tried to gain control over
the college curriculum, to strengthen the requirements, and to
lengthen the distance between portals of entrance and exit. Through
rigid licensing examinations it tried to establish still another process
of separating the fit from the unfit and of destroying institutions that
produced the latter. Through the creation of single licensing boards
it attempted to regulate rival schools of healing and to circumscribe
their work. In an effort to destroy the jungle of state statutes regulat-

ing medical licensure and practice it proposed uniform laws and measures to promote reciprocity among the states.

COUNCIL ON MEDICAL EDUCATION CREATED

When the AMA created the Council on Medical Education in June 1904, the reform of medical education appeared to be all but hopeless. Medical schools in the United States numbered 166, or about one-half of the total in the entire world. But unlike the medical schools of Europe, American institutions had developed wholly unregulated by federal law and largely uncontrolled by state legislation. Nor did they subscribe to only one medical system, but supplied recruits for every major healing sect. Thirty-three of these institutions offered homeopathic, eclectic, or physiomedical instruction, while another propagated various forms of sectarian dogma.[4] Unable to endow the council with coercive powers, the AMA created an agency that could work only through the use of pressure and persuasion, which diminished somewhat as it sought to control irregular groups. It had abandoned as hopeless an idea that the *Journal* endorsed in 1901 calling for the establishment of a national bureau of health and medicine empowered to compile data on medical licensure, to regulate medical practice, and to recommend uniform statutes to state legislatures. Instead it established its own council, which it authorized to issue reports on the condition of medical education in the United States and to make recommendations to the AMA on educational policies.[5]

The council, composed of men of exceptional talent, lost no time in beginning its work. Holding three conferences at Philadelphia in December 1904, at Chicago in April 1905, and at Portland three months later, it formulated immediate objectives for the improvement of medical education that the House of Delegates at its annual session in the latter year readily endorsed. To the Chicago conference it invited representatives of state examining and licensing boards and officials in government services and in colleges of liberal arts who assisted in developing goals for educational reform and in broadening the base of support for the program.[6]

COUNCIL'S FIRST OBJECTIVES

Committed to the idea of gradual reform, the council proposed at first only moderate objectives that it believed could be reached by 1

January 1908. Its plan set up as a preliminary requirement for medical school entrance a high school diploma or its equivalent and, according to an agreement reached at the Chicago conference, placed the validation of entrance requirements on state superintendents of education rather than on medical school authorities. It required that medical schools offer a four-year course of instruction of thirty weeks in a year and of thirty hours of actual work in a week, which met the total minimum demand of thirty-six hundred hours to which representatives at the Chicago conference had agreed.[7]

In formulating its plans the council did not conceal its desire for more stringent requirements that could not be realized immediately. It envisioned the establishment of a five-year curriculum of which the first year would be devoted to the study of physics, chemistry, and biology, either in a college of liberal arts or in a medical school. The following two years would be devoted primarily to the study of anatomy, physiology, pathology, and pharmacology, and the last two would include work with patients in dispensaries and hospitals in the study of such subjects as surgery and obstetrics. It also hoped to see the addition of a sixth-year internship as a prerequisite for practice[8] (see Appendix I).

COUNCIL'S EARLY WORK

The council's formulation of general rules for the improvement of medical training began its leadership of a movement for educational reform. It launched ambitious programs of its own and carried on other work that it inherited. It began to collect information on medical statutes in the states, the territories, and even in foreign countries. It gathered much material on the structure, powers, and operations of state boards of health. It sought information on the claims, standards, and practices of American medical schools. Among the inherited programs the most important was the collection, classification, analysis, and publication of statistical data on medical education that the *Journal* had begun in 1901. A year after the establishment of the council this publication struck its hardest blow at inferior medical institutions when it published the high failure rates of their students on state licensing board examinations. Based on the record of these graduates before licensing agencies, the council prepared its first rating of medical schools, grouping them into four classes. Through the pages of the *Journal* it continued to bring to light evidence that was damaging to the reputation of many medical schools. It also took on the important function of encouraging and coordinating the work of the forty-five committees on medical education that state and territorial medical associations had established by the spring of 1907.[9]

THE FIRST INSPECTION

The greatest work of the council had not yet begun. Well did it realize that statistical demonstrations could do little to improve or to destroy pretentious institutions resistant to reform. Nor could it rely on the Association of American Medical Colleges or any regional accrediting body to enforce standards that many medical schools persistently had ignored. Confronting the hostility of several institutions and restricted by limited finances, it launched a program for the inspection of all of the medical schools in the nation which no other agency or organization had ever dared to attempt.[10] The publicity that the press gave to a layman's classic survey of medical education four years later (the Flexner *Report* described herein) has done much to consign the council's pioneer work to undeserved obscurity.

The council made extensive plans for its investigation and decided to inspect not only regular medical schools but all of the homeopathic and eclectic institutions as well. It prepared a ten-point standard of inspection by which it tested the capacity of a school to offer acceptable medical education and by which it measured campus performance against catalog promise. It reviewed the total educational program, from the entrance requirements and their enforcement to the record of an institution's graduates on licensing board examinations. It inspected buildings, libraries, and laboratories; it investigated an institution's access to the facilities of hospitals and dispensaries, the extent of its reliance on full-time teachers in the first two years of instruction, and the extent of their opportunity for research. It also sought to discover whether a school existed largely for financial profit of the faculty or for the advancement of medical education[11] (see Appendix II).

Using the ten-point standard, the council developed a descending scale of ratings that ranged from A to F. Allowing a maximum of 10 percent for the rating of a college on any one of the ten points of measurement it gave a rating of A to colleges that scored 90 or above. It assigned a B rating to colleges scoring between 80 and 90; C to institutions scoring between 70 and 80; D to institutions falling between 60 and 70; and E to schools falling in the next decentile.

Institutions that dropped below 50 received the rating of F. It proposed to give recognition only to colleges that retained ratings of 70
or above, or that raised their ratings to that level, and contended that
only such institutions should be recognized by state boards of health.[12]

In the fall of 1906 the council's inspection began. All members
shared in the work though only one visited each medical school,
usually accompanied by the secretary of the council, Nathan P. Colwell. Even though these visits held out the prospect of severe criticism, officials of most colleges extended a cordial welcome and made
no effort to obstruct the work. Only rarely did authorities of local
schools put up a front of defiance. Before leaving on a trip to inspect
the schools of Louisville, however, Arthur D. Bevan and Colwell were
asked to stay away. Ignoring the warning, they went to Louisville and
found the officials somewhat subdued and even hospitable. Undoubtedly the discretion exercised by the investigators and their understanding of the problems of struggling institutions greatly reduced the
development of friction.[13] But the situation they explored sorely taxed
their capacity for patience and restraint. Weak and worthless institutions outnumbered better ones. Even in the most reputable institutions the council, to its surprise, found serious inadequacies, while
weaker ones often had virtually no foundations on which to build.
Years later Colwell described his inspection of some of the inferior
schools to a conference of secretaries of constituent state medical
associations, saying that had they accompanied him on his tour they
would have pitied patients exposed to the treatment of their graduates.
One school, he reported, that produced 105 graduates in 1905 had
neither a bottle in its laboratory nor a patient in its hospital or dispensary, and Bevan cited institutions with no laboratories at all.[14]
Some schools had no hospital or dispensary for clinical instruction,
and the connection in others with these auxiliary units was far from
satisfactory. Even the Yale Medical School had no hospital under its
control, and William T. Councilman reported that on his inspection
he found estrangement between the two institutions and the eighteen
beds assigned to the school wholly inadequate.[15]

When its survey was completed the council tabulated its data and
published its conclusions. The often sketchy and inaccurate information that medical schools formerly had submitted was replaced by
vast accumulations of more objective data. Even with the council's
moderate standard of evaluation, only eighty-one institutions received

ratings of 70 or above. Forty-seven lay within the range from 50 to 70, and thirty-two fell below the 50 mark. Thus the council found that one-half of the medical schools maintained tolerable standards, nearly one-third had an unacceptable but not hopeless rating, while one-fifth had hardly any standards. Despite the council's effort to deal fairly with irregular schools, they usually rated low, though often distinctly better than some regular institutions.[16]

ALLIED INVESTIGATIONS

Committees on medical education of several state societies supported the survey of the council of the AMA with investigations of their own. In June 1907 a committee of the Illinois society reported that it had completed an investigation of all of the medical colleges in the state and planned to publish an account of its findings. The same year, John T. Moore, chairman of the inspection committee of the Texas association, reported that he had investigated all but one of the medical schools of the state and that the graduates of less than half of them deserved recognition before the state licensing board. Allowing no school to escape inspection, the state association appointed a committee to make a special investigation of a notorious institution in Texarkana that for some undisclosed reason Moore had missed. So great was the association's growing pressure on inferior schools that three years later Moore reported the collapse of three institutions since his inspection began, but that even the four that remained created a surplus.[17]

The AMA's crusade for educational reform also derived considerable support from government agencies in some states. The Missouri State Board of Health gave special aid to the council's work. It appointed a committee from its own membership to investigate all of the medical schools in the state to determine which could be classified as reputable, an action justified by the opinion of the attorney general that it had the power to make such classifications and to exclude graduates of disreputable institutions from the examinations of the state licensing board. Soon some of the weaker institutions of the state that long had functioned largely without restraint were forced to reform or to perish, and not all could choose the former course.[18]

Although Pennsylvania joined late in the effort to advance educational reform, it created a Bureau of Medical Education and Licensure in 1911 that soon concluded the only thorough appraisal of medical schools ever made in the state. Thus, from Illinois and Missouri, where some of the most deplorable conditions in medical education prevailed, to at least one state with a more favorable record in the East, the AMA combined its power with that of state societies or government agencies, or both, to bring about reform. The success of the AMA's own work has largely obscured the extent of its reliance on government support. As early as 1908, its Council on Medical Education could report that twenty-nine states had given their examining boards full authority to deny recognition to colleges failing to meet prescribed standards and that boards in two other states held limited powers of recognition.[19]

The completion of the inspection gave the council no idea that its work had ended, but instead greater determination to proceed. Within a year it had "confirmed" its findings by checking on medical schools in fourteen states. This investigation more than confirmed former judgments; it provided evidence for rating eight more colleges beneath the 50 mark. Furthermore, it allowed members of the council to establish a closer alliance with state examining boards whose representatives usually accompanied them on inspection tours within their own states.[20]

WIDENING RESPONSIBILITIES

Its insistence on general reform in medical education quickly carried the work of the council beyond the stage of inspecting the schools. It could not call for standards in medical education that began with minimum admission requirements of a high school diploma and ignore the public educational structure beneath. By the fall of 1907, it had learned to its dismay that in eight southern and western states elementary and intermediate education consisted of only seven grades and that high schools in several of these states fell below the national four-year standard. The council appealed to leading educators in some of these states to support recommendations of the Committee of Ten of the National Education Association that called for the establishment of an eight-year elementary and intermediate school system and for four-year high schools, specifying the curriculum for the latter. It kept informed of progress that states had made toward these goals, reporting to the National Education Association on plans in Virginia and Texas to increase the number of four-year high schools.[21]

Direct reform of medical education remained, of course, the council's major goal, and the interim between the inspection of 1906–7 and another it conducted two years later was especially important in advancing constructive policies. In bringing together the largest body of data on medical education that the medical profession ever assembled in the United States, the council provided invaluable service to countless administrators, agencies, and groups that sought its aid. During this period it made the annual conferences on medical education (dating from 1904) a mighty instrument of reform as college administrators and representatives of state examining and licensing boards and of federal agencies united their efforts more closely for common goals. Furthermore, its appointment of a Committee of One Hundred, consisting of prominent educators, to draft a national uniform medical curriculum meant that it had replaced the sketchy guidelines it had offered medical schools with a comprehensive plan.[22] The curriculum that the council pressed medical schools to adopt after 1909 contributed greatly to the advance of educational reform in the second decade.

THE SEARCH ABROAD

In still other ways the two years after the first inspection brought notable developments. The council's thinking matured as its members reckoned with problems lying beyond the narrow range of curriculum reform. The efforts of many schools to adopt its recommendations clearly revealed the inadequacy of its program by showing that curriculum changes and physical improvements could not bring new vigor and life to enfeebled institutions. In drafting its earlier recommendations the council had followed some of the patterns in English and German schools. Again it turned abroad, not as much for procedural insights as to capture the more elusive qualities of the academic spirit. Seeking more accurate information on foreign medical education, it sent Colwell on a tour in 1908 that involved study of medical schools in nineteen European and South American countries.[23]

While awaiting Colwell's report, Bevan searched for the qualities that accounted for the greatness of some of the European medical schools. He traced much of the weakness of medical education in the United States to inferior instruction, considering the problem, next to that of raising medical school entrance requirements, as probably the greatest one facing the profession. He observed that all too often laboratory courses were taught by instructors who had never completed

medical training or by physicians devoting most of their time to private practice. He urged that laboratory instruction be rescued from
carelessness and neglect and cited the German plan of training professors for clinical instruction as approaching the ideal. Furthermore,
he deplored the estrangement that often developed between laboratory and clinical instructors and a tendency of the former to believe
that they alone taught scientific medicine. Quoting with approval a
statement of the great German internist, Friedrich Mueller, who contended that bedside observations should be given as high scientific
status as observations on animals, Bevan called for greater collaboration among laboratory and clinical instructors, citing the scientific
departments of Rudolf Virchow, Wilhelm Waldeyer, Robert Koch, and
others as examples of the success of such cooperation.[24]

Bevan called for the improvement of clinical instruction but not
along some of the lines often recommended. Citing the difficulty of
attracting a twenty-five-thousand-dollar man to a twenty-five-hundred-
dollar post, he opposed advocates of full-time clinical appointments
by showing the advantages of employing able part-time clinicians who
continued to engage in private practice. The work of Theodor Billroch
and Theodor Kocher in Germany and of Nicholas Senn and Christian
Fenger in the United States attested, he believed, to the superiority
of combining clinical instruction with private practice. Again, following the German model, he urged the recruitment to clinical posts of
men with experience in laboratory instruction and research. Adoption
of such a policy, he contended, not only would improve the quality of
training but would promote greater cooperation between laboratory
and clinical departments of medical schools.[25]

THE SECOND INSPECTION

As the council explored the larger dimensions of medical education
at the close of the decade it also conducted a second general inspection of medical schools. Responding to the influx of Canadian physicians into the United States, it reviewed all of the medical institutions of Canada. Again it used the ten-point standard (only slightly
modified) and prepared a list of 25 points called "Essentials of An
Acceptable Medical College" that served as a more specific measurement of institutional conditions (see Appendix III). Although it
expanded the grading scale from 100 to 1,000 points, it continued to
report college ratings in percentages. Making only three classifications,

it rated seventy-eight institutions (seventy-four American) above 70 percent in Class A; thirty-four (thirty-one American) between 70 and 50 percent in Class B; and thirty-two (thirty-one American) below 50 percent in Class C. The council considered Class A colleges as acceptable; Class B as in need of specific improvements; and Class C as colleges that needed complete reorganization for approval. For the first time it published the ratings of institutions by name in the *Journal* and extended the publicity with the issuance of more than five thousand reprints by June 1910.[26]

THE COUNCIL'S RECORD

Publication of the second report marks the end of a notable era in the council's history. In contrast to its work throughout the second decade, the achievements of the first decade may be attributed largely to its own efforts. Its attack on substandard schools had reduced the total number of medical institutions from 166 in 1904 to 136 in 1910, with 27 of the 30 merging or collapsing during the interval between the publication of reports on the two inspections.[27] Thus, from the time of its establishment, the council had largely brought about the collapse or merger of over 18 percent of the nation's medical schools, over 14 percent of them after the report of the first inspection. Undoubtedly, publication of the second report hastened the collapse or merger of many more. Striking at some of the most deplorable centers of educational chaos, it placed eight medical colleges in Illinois, seven in Missouri, and six in Tennessee in Class B or C. Eight of the seventeen surviving homeopathic institutions got similar ratings, while five of the remaining eclectic schools fell in Class C.[28] Such a record amply attests to the actual and potential effectiveness of its work.

But the council had scored other victories. Moving away from insistence on only a high school education as a prerequisite for medical training, the council, in its "Essentials of An Acceptable Medical College," called for a minimum requirement of "at least one year's college work" largely in specified sciences "as soon as conditions warrant." It reported that by the fall of 1910 two-thirds of the "acceptable" medical schools would require a year of college work largely given over to the study of biology, physics, and chemistry, and that sixteen Class A institutions required two or more years of college training. It also noted that ten other schools planned to require two years of college

work by the beginning of the following fall semester and that at least
six medical schools offered an optional fifth year of hospital training.
Furthermore, the council reported substantial improvement in state
board requirements of preliminary education. Boards in twenty-three
states prohibited medical schools from accepting students who had
not completed four years of high school training while seven other
boards required one or more years of college work.[29]

THE FLEXNER REPORT

Just as the publication of the council's report on the second inspection in June 1910 closed an era of reform in medical education, the
publication of the Flexner *Report* a few weeks earlier heralded the
opening of another. Well before the council could anticipate the success of its reform effort and fearful that its own resources were inadequate for the task, it appealed for assistance to Henry S. Pritchett,
president of the Carnegie Foundation for the Advancement of Teaching. Pritchett was sympathetic to the request and in 1908 persuaded a
layman, Abraham Flexner (brother of Simon Flexner, director of the
Rockefeller Institute for Medical Research), to undertake what would
pass as an outside survey of medical education, ostensibly disinterested and detached. Flexner's qualifications for the task included his
study of several colleges in England and France, investigation of some
of Germany's hospitals and nursing schools, and research upon which
he based his first book, *The American College.*[30]

About a half-century later Flexner confessed to his ignorance of medical education and to a feeling of inadequacy as he began his work.
But he approached his task with apparent confidence, beginning his
survey with an inspection of the Tulane School of Medicine in New
Orleans in January 1909. By March 1910, after devoting ten months
to the inspection, he had practically completed his investigation of 155
medical schools and postgraduate institutions in the United States and
Canada and had prepared his volume for publication. It reached the
public almost immediately after the inspection ended. Newspapers
hastily publicized his "pitiless" exposure, which, according to Flexner,
"produced an immediate and profound sensation."[31]

Actually, Flexner's *Report* struck citadels of medical instruction
with the force of a tornado and left many medical educators stunned
and shocked. Many old and venerable institutions swayed before his
attack, while scores of weaker schools were all but uprooted. Offering

a separate report on every school, he made specific and often damaging charges, preventing institutions from escaping the impact of his censure through anonymity. Of the two schools in Arkansas he said that "neither has a single redeeming feature," and he found it "incredible that the state university should permit its name to shelter one of them." Of the Georgia College of Eclectic Medicine and Surgery he charged that "nothing more disgraceful calling itself a medical school can be found anywhere." He described six Missouri schools as "utterly wretched" and three others as "feeble and without promise."[32] He found the dissecting room of the Kansas Medical College, that served also as a chicken yard, "indescribably filthy." At the Pacific College of Osteopathy he reported that students were "drilled to treat gonorrhea by diet and antiseptics" and "syphilis with ointments and dietetics." In the District of Columbia he contended that neither the Georgetown University School of Medicine nor the George Washington Department of Medicine could properly train modern physicians, and of the medical schools in Chicago, he asserted that "Rush alone is secure" on its admission policy and that none provided adequate clinical materials.[33]

Flexner exposed not only deficiencies in specific institutions, but basic weaknesses in the entirety of medical education. He considered a system of education substantially maintained by proprietary institutions wholly indefensible, particularly when such schools operated solely for profit. Some of the greatest educational abuses existed in proprietary and sectarian schools, and Flexner considered no abuse greater than minimal admission requirements that all too often gave way to an acceptance of their "equivalent." When school authorities exercised the right to accept an equivalent as a substitute for their own low standards, they really had, insisted Flexner, no standards at all.[34]

FLEXNER REPORT ATTACKED

The scathing attack on medical education brought instant protests and reprisals. Flexner received anonymous letters threatening his life and assurances of libel suits; officials of the St. Louis College of Physicians and Surgeons were so enraged by his assault that they filed a $100,000 damage suit against him, Colwell, and George H. Simmons.[35] Writers in sectarian medical journals, officials in irregular medical schools, and other sectarian spokesmen made bitter outcries, and

vehement protests rose from other sources. Some authorities in regular medical institutions censured by Flexner quickly struck back, and
an occasional distinguished and detached conventional physician
challenged the findings of the survey. Several university presidents and
lay educators who feared the growing dominance of American education by private foundations warned of that danger.

Homeopathic leaders concealed none of their resentment toward
Flexner, Pritchett, Bevan, and the Council on Medical Education.
Already a spokesman for homeopathy had denounced the "Czar-like
methods" of Bevan at the February meeting of the council and allied
groups. James R. Horner, in an editorial in the *Journal of the American
Institute of Homeopathy*, condemned Flexner's effort to reform medical education "in one fell swoop" as "suicidal" and "almost criminal."
The *Clinical Report* observed that modesty had no place "in the cate-
gory of his virtues" and that his positiveness was hardly justified either
by his eminence or by his authority, unless "authority is to flow from
an unlimited access to the pocketbook of a millionaire."[36] In September 1910 the Homeopathic Medical Society of the State of New York
caustically denied his charges about the obsolescence of its system.
Two months later the official organ of the movement denounced the
Carnegie Foundation for the "fruit of its labor" in Iowa where fresh-
man enrollment in the three medical schools (one homeopathic)
dropped 80 percent after the foundation had induced the schools to
adopt a two years of college requirement.[37]

Even louder protests came from some irregular institutions that
were major targets of attack. John K. Scudder, editor of the *Eclectic
Medical Journal,* charged that the major goal of the Carnegie and
Rockefeller interests was the economic advancement of the profession
through reduction of physician supply and state university control
over recruitment. Behind the conspiracy to seize control of medical
education, he insisted, lurked the AMA, which not only sought to
control the prescription policies of the profession through the Council
on Pharmacy and Chemistry, but to dominate medical education by
taking over supervisory functions that state boards of health or similar agencies normally assumed. W. T. Webster had the AMA's agitation for a national health department in mind when he spoke a few
months later of its sinister effort to extend its control over medical
practice from the state to the federal level.[38] George W. Thompson
warned the AMA in his presidential address of 1910 that "the enemy"

had struck at eclectic colleges in an effort to destroy the system and that "greedy capital," which had made American workers "victims of plunder," now hoped to subjugate the medical profession. The editor of the *Journal of the American Osteopathic Association* charged that the *Report* slandered osteopathic schools and that "the mean bitterness and bigotry of the inspection is evident in almost every sentence," particularly when it dealt with institutions other than "allopathic colleges."[39]

Groups of physicians and individual doctors made scattered protests. The Council on Medical Education of the Missouri State Medical Association cited disparities between Flexner's appraisals and the ratings of the Council on Medical Education of the AMA. It noted that Flexner called the University Medical College in Kansas City "utterly wretched" while the AMA's council gave it a rating of A and that two other schools in the state that Flexner denounced in similar fashion received B ratings from the council. George W. Webster, head of the Illinois State Board of Health, cited the incredible haste with which Flexner conducted his survey, while Henry C. Tinkham, dean of the University of Vermont College of Medicine, deplored the impact of the report on small schools. George R. West, dean of the Chattanooga Medical College, protested to the editor of *Collier's* for publishing an article allegedly full of errors and distortions in which Flexner attacked his school, adding that "Mr. Flexner condemned our railroads as he arrived, our hotels as he tarried, and our medical colleges as he passed on." George H. Stover, dean of the Denver and Gross College of Medicine, complained to Andrew Carnegie that within five minutes of an interview he saw that Flexner was decidedly prejudiced "*before* he made even a prefunctory 'inspection.' "[40] But the sharpest criticism came from G. Frank Lydston, a prominent physician of Chicago. Referring to officials of the AMA as "impertinent porcine trust-monopolists," he said of Flexner: "That in his entire tour of meddling with other people's business, the lay volunteer inspector of medical colleges was not once refused admission, kicked down the front steps, is a reflection on medical manhood."[41]

From abroad, the renowned William Osler of Oxford University wrote in a confidential report to the president of the Johns Hopkins University (where he had served on the medical faculty) that the Flexner survey, as it appeared, never should have been published and that the author made mistakes that no layman could have avoided.

Osler resented Flexner's criticism of the clinical staff of the institution and objected to Flexner's emphasis on the employment of full-time clinicians and to some of his proposals for reorganizing the school.[42]

Criticisms of the Flexner *Report* represented in part a suspicion of Carnegie and Rockefeller philanthropy that mounted rapidly in the second decade. The public properly joined the two groups in its attack, for Carnegie retained membership on the General Education Board for ten years after his appointment in 1908, while Flexner continued to exert a dominant influence through much of this period.[43] The "massacre" of twenty helpless strikers and children at Ludlow, Colorado, on 20 April 1914 by remnants of the Colorado National Guard, dominated by the Rockefeller-controlled Colorado Fuel and Iron Company, cast further doubt on the design of Rockefeller munificence. Fearing the damage of such publicity, the Rockefeller interests selected the rising public relations expert, Ivy Ledbetter Lee, to assist in removing additional tarnish from its name.[44]

A decade after Carnegie had set up his college pension fund, some leading educational spokesmen considered his gesture less noble than altruism. In 1914, when John E. Churchill, president of the Board of Education of New York, charged that the foundation stood as a "menace to the freedom of teaching" and called for its dissolution, William Oxley Thompson and Alston Ellis, presidents respectively of the Ohio State University and the University of Ohio, agreed with his criticism and warned of the controls that Carnegie philanthropy sought to impose.[45] The National Education Association, disturbed by the danger, likewise issued a strong protest: "We view with alarm the activity of Carnegie and Rockefeller foundations; agencies not in any way responsible to the people, in their efforts to control the policies of our state educational institutions; to fashion after their conception and to standardize our course of study, and to surround the institutions with conditions which menace true academic freedom and defeat the primary purpose of democracy as heretofore preserved inviolate in our common schools, normal schools and universities."[46]

The famous *Report* that brought censure upon Flexner and the Carnegie and Rockefeller empires brought praise and acclaim as well. Naturally the *Journal* of the AMA lost no opportunity to extol the survey. Organs of state societies usually responded with more than ritualistic tribute. The *Ohio State Medical Journal* reflected the general sentiment of these publications when it called the study a product of "painstaking labor" and added, "The report will, we are confident, serve the high purpose of the Foundation in promoting the progress of medical education, and to this end we bespeak for it careful study from cover to cover by every one who is in any way charged with the responsibility of managing medical colleges in this country."[47]

Both favorable and adverse appraisals of the Flexner *Report* contained a considerable measure of truth. The survey's attack on the unscientific aspects of medical education fell far short of the scientific standards Flexner sought to impose. Flexner's haste in inspecting in a period of three months sixty-nine medical schools in twenty-two states in not more than seventy-eight working days raises serious questions.[48] Numbered among these institutions were substantial and thriving schools requiring careful inspection as well as ones that could be rather casually dismissed as deficient and infirm. What account did Flexner take of the plans of some of the latter for the improvement of their facilities and faculties and of the efforts that many institutions made to meet the early recommendations of the AMA's educational council? What appreciation did he show for the contributions of some sectarian systems that, in resisting the medical nihilism of the regular profession, preserved faith in the possibilities of therapeutic advance? Why did he seek to impose on medical students a scientific regimen that practically excluded ethical and cultural approaches to their own profession? Why did he send tentative drafts of his impressions to some of the better schools for their correction while apparently offering no opportunity to many weaker institutions to correct his misapprehensions and mistakes?[49] Yet, whatever its limitations, the Flexner survey accelerated the movement for educational reform which the American Medical Association already had well under way. Flexner sought to reduce physician supply and to raise the standards of medical education, and the former goal was not incidental to the latter. Accordingly, his survey must be interpreted as both an economic and a scientific work, receiving an acclaim only partially deserved.[50]

NEW DIRECTIONS

In the year 1910 two eras of educational reform merged and momentum was provided for the progress of the second decade. Private philanthropy, as represented by the Carnegie Foundation for the Advancement of Teaching and by Rockefeller's General Education Board, supplemented the work of the AMA as its Council on Medical Education kept up the struggle to raise standards. This agency now stressed the higher objectives of its twenty-five-point program (later twenty-six), calling for one year of college work and possibly for even two as a prerequisite for medical study, and it began to insist on a year's internship as a requirement for practice though it had referred to this innovation in its recommendations of 1905.[51] The Carnegie Foundation and the General Education Board seemed more demanding because they encouraged medical schools to adopt a two-year entrance requirement and supported plans for the establishment of full-time clinical positions in medical colleges. By advocating the two-year entrance standard the board and the foundation employed means to make the plan palatable to a number of medical schools before the council could free itself from a tacit obligation to support simply the one-year goal. By subsidizing experiments for the employment of full-time clinicians the board pioneered in trying to advance another unpopular scheme.

PRESSURES OF PHILANTHROPY

Although the council carried the burden of the struggle in the second decade, the Carnegie Foundation for the Advancement of Teaching sought to impose the two-year entrance requirement by denying to schools that failed to comply the benefit of its faculty pension subsidy. In 1915, Simon P. Kramer, a professor in the Medical School of the University of Cincinnati, complained of the confusion in his state where the law required a high school certificate for medical school entrance, while the Council on Medical Education insisted on one year of college and the Carnegie Foundation on two. He traced the strength of the latter requirement to the $750,000 which the foundation had distributed in pension subsidies among institutions that met its demands.[52]

In supporting a movement for the employment of full-time clinicians in medical schools the General Education Board hoped to achieve substantial reform in clinical research and instruction. Responding to an appeal from William H. Welch in 1913 for the establishment of endowed chairs in medicine, pediatrics, and surgery in the Department of Medicine at the Johns Hopkins University, it launched its pioneer experiment with income from a $1.5 million grant to that institution and raised a dispute over the merits of the plan that out-lasted the decade.[53]

This innovation brought up several issues that became more serious when other schools sought resources for similar programs. Some medical educators believed that a system employing a part-time clinical staff, continually improved by experience in private practice, attracted the ablest talent and offered the greatest hope for the improvement of clinical medicine. They also thought that few medical schools could bear the added cost of such programs, which required greater remuneration for clinicians deprived of supplementary sources of income. Furthermore, they reminded proponents of such plans that the reserves schools acquired from the work of clinical departments often would place disproportionate burdens on the ablest members of their staffs.[54]

Disturbed by the growing emphasis on full-time clinical appointments, the Council of Medical Education selected a committee to investigate the merits of the issue. In February 1915, the committee "practically endorsed" the proposed policy after consultation with educators of varying views. The council, however, showed no immediate intention of following such a course since Bevan, chairman both of the council and of the more innovative committee, remained an outspoken critic of the plan. Four years after the Progressive Era ended he contended that the proposal never secured the support of the medical profession and that all of the rare experiments with full-time clinical positions had failed.[55]

THE THIRD INSPECTION

Having passed through a triumphal epoch in educational reform by the close of 1910, the council sought the realization of its higher academic goals and refused to be diverted by what it regarded as peripheral issues. It had no reason to question the verdict of the AMA's *Journal* in 1911 that the profession was still "seriously overcrowded" and that many medical schools could not provide an adequate medical course.[56] It prepared for another inspection of schools the following year to measure the progress of educational reform and the remaining resistance to its work.

The council considered the 120 medical schools it inspected in 1912 still too many, though 16 had passed away through merger or extinction in the last two years. Regretfully, it reported that at least 45 colleges held onto admission standards requiring less than a high school education. It noted that only 33 had close connections with universities and that 56 had made no provision for medical research. Only about 30 medical schools in the United States, it concluded, ranked with medical institutions of advanced nations abroad. On the brighter side, the council noted that 16 medical schools had admission requirements calling for one year of college work and that 30 others required two years or more. It also reported that nine state licensing boards had a one- or two-year college requirement. It claimed that the profession faced three tasks: securing agreement among licensing boards on the amount of education required for medical practice; reorganizing medical departments after the German plan that provided for the training of competent teaching staffs; and establishing a closer connection between medical schools and charity hospitals.[57]

Clearly concentrating on objectives that appeared more readily attainable, the council followed the third inspection with principal stress on the internship problem and on an admission standard requiring one year of college work. In emphasizing an internship the council could not escape responsibility for investigating hospitals in which interns served. Early in 1913 it canvassed 2,424 of the nation's hospitals with twenty-five beds or more and received replies from 2,185. Of these it found that only 852, or only 39 per cent, made regular use of interns. Upon the validation of information supplied by hospitals to committees of physicians, which it had appointed in every state, the council issued an approved list of hospitals for internship training in 1914. The following year it persuaded state societies to establish permanent committees for hospital evaluation, and in 1916 it issued a revised list of hospitals acceptable for internships after examining returns from a second questionnaire. This list provided prospective interns with their only guide in selecting hospitals.[58]

As the council laid the foundation for internship programs it achieved more immediate results through its insistence on the one-year college standard. The haste with which other institutions raised admission standards partially attested to the growing emphasis the council had placed on college training for admission. World War I had just begun when it announced that fifty-two colleges already required one or more years of college work and that twenty-three others would be added to the list within a year, increasing the total to seventy-five. It watched many weak institutions that somehow had survived in the educational upheaval collapse before its growing pressure. When in

1915 only ninety-five schools remained (a drop of twenty-five in three years), the achievement of the crusade appears all the more impressive. Medical school enrollments that reached 28,142 in the year the council was created fell to about one-half that number (14,891) in 1915.[59]

As the Progressive Era closed the council reported statistics that revealed the success of its appeal to state boards for higher standards of admission. In forty-four states the health boards or comparable agencies set at least a high school education as the minimum admission requirements to medical schools within their jurisdictions. But thirty-six of these required at least one year of college work and twenty-one set a two-year minimum. In 1916, when the council decreed that all medical institutions must establish a two-year college entrance requirement by 1 January 1918 to receive a Class A rating, it sealed the fate of other struggling schools. Forty-two state boards had power to deny recognition to institutions that could not meet these standards and six of these required internships for medical practice.[60]

The tangible goals that the AMA and philanthropic foundations achieved in less than one and a half decades of struggle somewhat obscure other ominous and far-reaching goals. The success of their warfare on many private schools cast the burden of medical education increasingly upon state institutions where many authorities conceded that it properly belonged. But as the burden shifted, medical leaders capitalized on public apathy relating to matters of health and medicine that they formerly and frequently had deplored and exposed. The public increasingly assumed the financial burden of the profession's training, but entrusted direction of health and medical policies to private medical associations over which it exercised almost no control. Even as the burden of medical education fell increasingly on the state, the will of the profession in an even larger measure became public policy. Portentous threats to general welfare appeared as public control and public finance of medical education operated in inverse ratio. Policies of negativism and restraint that medical leaders introduced in one era could prove disastrous in another. The success of the profession's effort to establish public policy required not only control of medical education, but demanded an alliance with the law as well. An account of the development and operation of this alliance is now in order.

CHAPTER FOUR

ALLIANCE WITH THE LAW

Even before the American Medical Association launched its program for the reform of medical education, its leadership had concluded that no amount of organizational exertion could substitute for government action in elevating the status and standards of the profession. Charles A. L. Reed aptly reflected growing acceptance of this position in his presidential address to the St. Paul session of the AMA in 1901. Maintaining that the gains of statutory regulation of medical practice in the last quarter of the nineteenth century stood in sharp contrast to the failure of the prescriptive policies of the profession and its efforts at self-regulation before that time, he called upon regular physicians to advance the movement for the effective exercise of political controls: "The legislative functions have passed from voluntary organizations to the Congress and the legislatures, where they belong; but it still devolves upon the profession in the organized capacity, to stimulate, to restrain, or otherwise to control the lawmaking power. The responsibility of the profession is increased, rather than diminished."[1]

POLITICAL GOALS

The formulation, enactment, strengthening, and protection of medical legislation became principal goals of the AMA and its constituent societies during the Progressive Era. Just as important, the national organization and its affiliates sought to establish and strengthen government agencies endowed with power to enforce legislation, accomplishing for the profession what it could not achieve through its own efforts. Spokesmen for the dominant profession rejoiced as much over the strengthening of a state licensing statute as over the collapse of a feeble medical school. In fact, they worked harder to accomplish the former than the latter for the advancement and protection of medical legislation, unlike the struggle for educational improvement, required that they secure effective support from medical organizations in every state.

HEALING GROUPS EMERGING

The multiplication of healing sects and groups late in the nineteenth century made the medical profession's concern for improved medical statutes all the more urgent. As the profession well knew, these irregular groups threatened to perpetuate in the new century much of the chaos of the old. From its headquarters in Boston the Christian Science movement steadily gained in followers and respectability and, to the dismay of regular physicians, had considerable success in removing the causes of disease out of their domain of practice and into the imagination. While troubled by the advance of this movement promoting psychic formulas for combating the alleged fantasy of disease, conventional physicians watched almost helplessly the emergence of osteopathy, which located most human ailments in the spinal column. Hardly had this sect appeared when the chiropractic system arose to challenge both their healing principles and osteopathic procedures. Optometrists moved in on an area preempted but neglected by the regular profession, and physiomedical and electrotherapeutic groups tempted the public with the novelty and diversity of their techniques. Early in the new century the influence of Dowieism survived among converts to the faith-healing ideas of John Alexander Dowie, who lived until 1907, while the theories of Elwood Worcester and Samuel McComb, organizers of the Emmanuel Movement in Boston, found receptivity among growing numbers increasingly susceptible to the psychic approach to most problems of disease.[2]

The struggle against emerging sects consumed much of the energies of the regular profession in the Progressive Era. Finding greatest danger in the spread of Christian Science, osteopathy, chiropractic, and optometry, the profession sought legislation to stop their encroachment on medical practice. All of these groups had made substantial headway before the twentieth century began, and more than two decades of growth lay behind the Christian Science movement that sprang from the teachings of Mary Baker Glover (later Eddy), who

published her views in *Science and Health* in 1875 and chartered the
first congregation of her followers in Boston four years later.[3] In attacking the foundations of medical practice and in developing considerable skill in securing exemption from medical practice statutes, the
movement gave the profession cause for considerable alarm even
before 1900.

Osteopathy presented a much graver threat when Andrew T. Still,
claiming to have taken a course at the Kansas City School of Physicians and Surgeons in the 1860s and tracing the formulation of his
theories to 22 June 1874, established the American School of Osteopathy at Kirksville, Missouri, in 1892. The founding of the National
School of Osteopathy and Infirmary Association in 1895, the Northern
School of Osteopathy, and the Pacific School of Osteopathy and Infirmary a year later gave the movement a formidable appearance at a
time when its success in securing legislative recognition in Vermont
in 1896 and in Missouri the following year bestowed upon it some
legal respectability.[4] Encouraged by the outcome of recent legislative
struggles, Still established what soon became the American Osteopathic Association. This organization spread the theories of the movement in the *Popular Osteopath,* a publication that expired in two
years, but served as a forerunner of the *Journal of the American
Osteopathic Association* that appeared in September 1901.[5]

Like Christian Science, osteopathy repudiated fundamental medical
concepts and was only slightly more generous than the religious sect to
conventional practitioners in conceding the necessity for occasional
recourse to major surgery that might require their services. Founders
of both groups claimed divine sanction for their mission, and in 1902,
Still wrote, "I quote no authors but God and experience."[6] Books
composed by medical authorities could be of little use, he contended,
in the propagation of a science they know nothing about. He defined
osteopathy as "a scientific knowledge of anatomy and physiology in
the hands of a person of intelligence and skill who can apply that
knowledge to the use of man when sick or wounded by strains, shocks,
falls, or mechanical derangement or injury of any kind to the body."[7]
Denying charges that osteopaths were only masseurs, he contended
that the latter made no use of any osteopathic principle. While assert-
ing that osteopathy recognized the validity of the germ theory in
explaining the origin of some diseases, he maintained that germs were
usually a secondary factor and that they could not infect the tissue

of a healthy body. In 1902 the *Journal of Osteopathy*, another publication of the movement, stated that it opposed the employment of drugs "as remedial agents," opposed use of vaccines and serums, and believed that "disease is the result of anatomical abnormalities followed by physiological discord." Furthermore, it contended that the house of healing was only large enough for osteopathy and that when other forms of practice entered, osteopathy had to move out.[8] Still expressed the movement's alienation from conventional physicians when he charged that they had erected "temples to the gods who purged, puked, perspired, opiated, drank whiskey and other stimulants," and he called for a war on these pretending healers and their surgical brethren as well.[9]

In 1899, when Still openly declared warfare on medical doctors, a rival movement dating from 1895 in an adjoining state also had been attacked by osteopaths. In opening an institution at Davenport, Iowa in 1897, Daniel D. Palmer launched himself and his chiropractic movement on a turbulent career. The distinctiveness of his system partially rested on his claim to have been the first person to replace dislocated vertebrae by using the "spinous and transverse process as levers."[10] While osteopathy related health to the "normal structural relationship" of the body, chiropractic theory traced most human ailments to the malfunctioning of the nervous system. Both groups employed manipulative techniques, but osteopaths deplored the alleged brutality of Palmer's assaults on the human body. Describing the adjustment methods demonstrated at the Davenport institution, a Los Angeles osteopath, Stanley M. Hunter, concluded, "Even Torquemada could hardly have invented, for the Spanish Inquisition a better method of extorting confessions."[11]

The chiropractic movement nevertheless pushed its way into the new century and received no great setback when its founder served a six-month jail term in 1903 for practicing medicine without a license. Bartlett J. Palmer, Daniel's son, took over the management of the institute, giving his father an opportunity, after the interim of enforced confinement, to fail twice in his efforts to establish a successful school in Portland, and once in Oklahoma City, before his retirement to private practice in 1907.[12] With only about one hundred practitioners, the movement established the Universal Chiropractors' Association in 1906, only four years before dissension between "straights" and "mixers" caused the latter to establish the National Chiropractic Association that brought together those who sometimes combined drugs, heat, light, water, electricity, and later vitamins with manipulative techniques in rendering treatment. The seventy-nine chiropractic schools that existed in 1920 attested little perhaps to the strength or popularity of the movement, but when chiropractors secured official recognition in Kansas in 1913, and a licensing law in Arkansas two years later, conventional physicians could no longer ignore their very real threat.[13]

Opticians heralded their efforts to secure legislative recognition of their trade early in the new century by employing the title "optometrist" to designate a member of their craft. But under whatever name they chose, they could not escape attacks from regular physicians who looked upon their efforts as an unwarranted invasion of a well-defined area of medical practice.[14] Opticians claimed that legislative recognition would prevent ill-trained and often itinerant glass fitters from preying on the public, but physicians discounted their argument as one designed to cut out disreputable tradesmen and medical specialists as well. David R. Silver, in his presidential address to the Ohio State Medical Association in 1909, expressed a common professional view when he charged that "optometry is the most plausible of any of the pretensions of quackery" and that it would indeed "deceive the very elect."[15]

Opticians added plausibility to their case when they cited the admitted failure of the medical profession to provide adequate training in eye refraction. In 1909 a prominent doctor, Leartus Conner, found that no more than 3,000 of the nation's 135,000 physicians (or only one in forty-five) could claim competency in refractive procedures. Another physician, James Thorington, traced the greatest incompetence in this type of practice to physicians trained before 1900, but insisted that the general negligence of the profession had allowed opticians to secure protective legislation.[16]

Yet professional ignorance and negligence only partially accounted for the gains of optometry in the new century. Disregarding the warnings of the medical profession, the public increasingly bypassed physicians who generally gave no more than prescriptions for opticians to fill and instead consulted optometrists who provided diagnosis, refraction, prescription, frames, and lenses. Nor could families struggling at the margin of poverty overlook the price advantage frequently offered by skilled tradesmen in eye refraction or the appeal of their advertisements.

SECTARIAN GROUPS ATTACKED

Against the growing ranks of the healing sects orthodox medical leaders conducted a two-fold offensive. They tried to impress the public with the fallacies and potential dangers of sectarian practice. On the political front they brought their case to the hearing rooms of legislative committees where sectarian groups often sought protection. But whether exposing the scientific fallacies of sectarian practitioners or countering their political strategy, orthodox leaders developed considerable skill in the Progressive Era. Reducing their arguments against cultism to laymen's language, they did much to diminish the appeal of the healing sects.

Orthodox medical spokesmen showed that cultism rested on simplistic notions about the causes and cures of infirmities and diseases. They deplored the fragmentation of the field of healing by sectarian groups that traced the origin of diseases to areas of their pretended competence. They showed that dogmatic healing systems by their very nature negated the scientific spirit that required adaptation to new medical discoveries and techniques. These systems, they contended, denied or only partially accepted such demonstrated facts as the bacteriological origin of many diseases. Sometimes physicians exposed what they looked upon as the curative deceptions of the healing cults. Charles A. L. Reed demonstrated this line of attack in the New York *Sun* just before the new century began when he offered to provide Mary Baker Eddy with advanced cases of cancer to heal, practically identical to a case that she claimed to have cured.[17]

Yet orthodox leaders did not confine their attacks to the theories and pretensions of the healing cults. They charged more frequently that sectarian practitioners were simply incompetent to treat human ailments and that sectarian schools seldom if ever taught the foundation courses in medical science. A Des Moines physician warned doctors in other states late in the Progressive Era of the alleged incompetence of graduates of Iowa's three chiropractic schools that offered no instruction in pharmacology, medicine, surgery, anesthesia, or embryology, that either did not teach at all or only from their sectarian view, bacteriology, gynecology, dermatology, and diseases of the eye, ear, nose, and throat, and that did not offer acceptable instruction in physiology and chemistry.[18] Regular medical leadership rated the training of osteopaths little if any higher and considered optometrists almost wholly incompetent in diagnosing and treating diseases of the eye.

In the sectarian struggles arising early in the Progressive Era orthodox physicians found it easier to define their purposes than their strategy. They wished to see single licensing boards established, composed
exclusively of regular physicians, guarding the only portal of entrance
into the profession. They hoped to control licensing boards by securing provisions in licensing laws confining appointments to lists of nom-
inees chosen by local societies. They hoped to reduce the hordes of
graduates that strong and weak medical schools alike poured into the
profession by securing legislation requiring that state licensing agencies examine every candidate.[19] They insisted on compulsory examinations and that each candidate present a diploma from a school the
board approved. They sought to strengthen statutory definitions of
medical practice to force on any person attempting to treat disease
compliance with the educational requirements of the statute. Furthermore, they tried to write professional ethics into legislation, bringing
the power of the state to the enforcement of ethical principles usually
inadequately enforced by local societies.

SINGLE BOARD STRATEGY

Despite an apparent commitment to rigid standards, orthodox
leaders often adopted a flexible strategy that subordinated major goals
to lesser gains. Although they had sought single licensing boards composed exclusively of regular physicians empowered to examine all
candidates for licensure, they sometimes could secure nothing nearer
to their liking than multiple boards or single boards on which sectarian groups had representation. By 1900 they had secured boards in
thirty-two states and continental territories (including the District of
Columbia) empowered to examine all candidates, but this achievement required concession in some instances to sectarian groups that
would accept nothing less than multiple or composite boards.[20]

The growth of the osteopathic and chiropractic movements caused
orthodox leaders to increase their agitation for single boards from
which representatives of these sects would be excluded, but they conceded representation of homeopaths and eclectics as a price for their
support. They conceded further by relaxing their insistence on the
selection of orthodox members of the board from a list recommended
by the state society when such a demand threatened to prevent enactment of regulatory legislation. In their struggle to bring irregular

groups under the requirements of the medical practice laws they usually agreed to exclude Christian Scientists rather than jeopardize passage of a bill. When unable to prevent enactment of legislation providing for the licensing of chiropractors, osteopaths, and optometrists, they sought rigorous statutory restrictions on their work to allow as little encroachment as possible on medical practice. When they found that they could not write many of their principles of medical ethics into law they preferred to concede rather than have their legislation defeated.

Issues involving the number, structure, and power of licensing boards created for the regular profession some of its hardest battles in the Progressive Era. The new laws enacted by legislatures of California, Kansas, Rhode Island, Missouri, Tennessee, and Texas in 1901 reflected the statutory chaos of the era and forecast the task before the profession. Orthodox physicians of California joined with homeopaths and eclectics in securing a composite board of nine members that included five regulars; in Kansas they accepted a composite board allowing no majority to any group; in Tennessee four regulars shared board positions with one eclectic and one homeopath; in Rhode Island three regulars served with one homeopath and three laymen. The Texas legislature yielded to the wishes of homeopaths and eclectics in creating three separate boards, and in Missouri the legislature kept examining and licensing functions within the state board of health, attempting to reconcile irregular groups with the provision that appointments could reflect no discrimination against the different medical systems.[21]

From 1900 to 1907 thirty state and territorial legislatures enacted new medical practice laws; these statutes varied greatly, but state medical societies imposed a measure of order on the drafting process. The secretary of the AMA's Council on Medical Education reported in April 1908 that New York, South Carolina, and Texas recently had replaced multiple with composite boards, leaving only ten states with two or more separate medical boards.[22] In the struggle for single boards state societies made further progress in the next decade. When the Progressive Era ended single boards had been established in forty-three states, twenty-six of which had single composite boards. Only five states and the District of Columbia retained multiple boards.[23]

The regular profession not only had experienced substantial success with its single boards strategy, but had scored other victories and preserved gains made late in the nineteenth century. Alabama, Maryland, and North Carolina entrusted the appointment of the board to the state medical society, and the medical practice laws of eleven other states and the District of Columbia specified that appointments must be made from a list chosen by state societies. While the laws of fourteen states specified that no system of medicine could have a majority of members on the board, twenty-nine states provided for single boards with no such restrictions.[24] (For the structure of medical boards at the end of the Progressive Era see Appendix IV.)

The regular profession used the single board strategy to establish actual or eventual dominance over the homeopathic and eclectic movements, but it had to find other methods to meet the threats raised by the emerging sects. Considering osteopathy and chiropractic as nothing more than quackery, it strongly opposed legal recognition of these groups.[25] It opposed representation of such sects on composite boards and resisted their efforts to secure separate boards. In fact, the regular profession fought its bitterest political battles in the Progressive Era against osteopaths over the separate board issue.

RESTRICTING CULT PRACTICE

In the struggle with osteopaths, orthodox medical leaders won substantial but only partial victories. Often unable to prevent the passage of laws creating separate boards, they succeeded only in securing in this legislation limitations on the boundaries of osteopathic practice. The Massachusetts law, for example, stipulated that "persons registering hereinunder shall not be permitted to prescribe or administer drugs for internal use, or to perform major operations in surgery, or to engage in the practice of obstetrics, or to hold themselves out, by virtue of such registration, as and for other than osteopaths."[26] With similar restrictions, seventeen states established osteopathic boards by 1910, and in ten others osteopaths had secured representation on state examining boards. By 1917 eighteen states had provided osteopaths with separate boards.[27]

Chiropractors, on the other hand, made no comparable advance. Only seven states followed Kansas after 1913 in licensing chiropractors before the Progressive period ended. As the era closed Christian Scientists had won specific exemptions from the medical practice laws in only ten states, and elsewhere the legality of much of their practice remained in doubt. Optometrists made more rapid gains, and over the opposition of opthalmologists they secured special licensing laws in thirty-nine states and two territories by 30 March 1917.[28]

LEGISLATING STANDARDS

Orthodox medical societies not only fought for single medical boards and for legislation restricting the boundaries of sectarian practice, but sought also a third major objective. They called for the enactment of laws prescribing the educational requirements of candidates for licensure and the nature of the examinations or for statutes conferring these powers on state examining boards. They wanted the states to deny examinations for licensure to graduates of institutions falling below standards specified by law or established by state boards. They sometimes secured legal specifications of courses on which all candidates would be tested, and in at least one instance, the passing grade level.[29]

Statutes varied, but a few examples of their provisions will indicate the influence of medical societies on the legislation in force near the end of the Progressive Era. Some laws recognized the standards prescribed by the American Association of Medical Colleges or by the Southern Association of Medical Colleges and excluded from examination graduates of institutions failing to meet these requirements.[30] The California law simply stipulated that a candidate must have attempted four courses of not less than thirty-two weeks in length and must have completed a total of four thousand class hours. Many states required that the applicant be a graduate of a "reputable" medical college, giving the board power to determine the standing of any school in question. The Texas law defined a "reputable school" as one whose standards were equal to the better class of medical schools in the nation.[31]

Regular societies contended that laws should require that all candidates for licensure pass tests in basic sciences whether or not they planned a career in regular medicine. In 1907 state boards required tests in an average of nine fields, varying from twenty-five in South Carolina to seven in Arkansas, Florida, and Maine. The tentative model medical practice act, drafted by a committee of the AMA in 1910, called for examination of all candidates in anatomy, chemistry, physiology, toxicology, pathology, symptomatology, surgery, and obstetrics, and many state statutes approximated these requirements. For irregular groups some states laid down extremely rigid demands. The Ohio law even required tests in anatomy, physiology, chemistry, bacteriology, hygiene, diagnosis, and "other subjects appropriate to the limited branches of medicine and surgery" of all who sought licenses to practice "chiropractic, napropathy, spondylotherapy, mechano-therapy, neuropathy, electro-therapy, hydrotherapy, suggestive-therapy, psycho-therapy, magnetic healing, chiropody, Swedish movements, massage," and other branches of medicine mentioned in the General Code except midwifery and osteopathy, only allowing specific exemption from tests in pathology and diagnosis for those practicing massage and Swedish movements.[32]

When regular medical organizations could not prevent the passage of osteopathic laws they sought to write rigid requirements into this legislation. The New Jersey law was not much more demanding than many others in requiring examinations in fifteen fields—anatomy, chemistry, physiology, pathology, toxicology, histology, hygiene, dietetics, gynecology, bacteriology, obstetrics, surgery, osteopathic and physical culture, the theory and practice of osteopathy, and medical jurisprudence. It also required that an applicant have a high school diploma or its equivalent and a diploma from a recognized osteopathic school that required three years of work. The New York law stipulated that the applicant have three specified sciences in high school, four years of training in a recognized osteopathic school, and pass board examinations in eight areas. Pennsylvania prescribed graduation from an osteopathic school requiring thirty-two months of work and examinations in at least eleven areas.[33] Regular medical societies did not believe that osteopathic boards would adhere very closely to their licensing laws, but they knew that a stringent measure was preferable to a weak one when the passage of some law seemed certain.

DEFINING MEDICAL PRACTICE

Still a fourth challenge faced the regular profession as it struggled for higher educational requirements, for legislation restricting the range of sectarian practice, and for single medical boards. Hoping to subject all healing sects to the demands and penalties of comprehensive medical practice laws, which prescribed standards they could barely if ever meet, it faced the tasks of defining the practice of medicine so as to include them all and of incorporating its definition into law. Yet despite the attention the profession gave the subject it could come to no agreement on a suitable definition of medical practice. A committee drafting a tentative law for the AMA in 1910 took more than three hundred words to define it, and this definition made little impression on state societies. In 1907 the definition of medical practice was comprehensive in the statute of the Arizona Territory, brief in the laws of Alabama, Connecticut, and Illinois, and nonexistent in nine states.[34] The medical practice act of the state of Washington provides perhaps the best example of a statute combining many features common to most of them:

Any person shall be deemed as practicing within the meaning of this act who shall have and maintain an office, or place of business with his or her name and the words physician or surgeon, "Doctor," "M.D." or "M.B." in public view, or shall assume or advertise the title of Doctor or any title which shall show or tend to show that the person assuming or advertising the same is a lawful practitioner of any of the branches of medicine or surgery in such a manner as to convey the impression that he or she is a practitioner of medicine or surgery under the laws of the state; or any person who shall practice medicine or surgery under a false or assumed name, or under cover of the name of some legal practitioner, or personate any legal practitioner, or for a fee, prescribe or direct, or recommend for the use of any person any drug or medicine for the treatment, care or relief of any wound, fracture or bodily injury, infirmity or disease.[35]

Healing sects often claimed immunity from medical regulation, contending that they did not engage in medical practice. The regular medical profession maintained that an essential feature of medical practice was diagnosis and that since all sects actually diagnosed, they practiced medicine. The profession contended that the administration of drugless therapy did not give cults immunity from medical practice statutes and that medical practice consisted of far more than drug treatment. So broad did the profession make the definition of medical practice in some state statutes that the laws frequently contained special clauses exempting such services as midwifery, "treatment by prayer," and the administration of domestic remedies (sometimes adding "without compensation" to the latter).[36] When the committee of the AMA prepared its tentative medical practice bill it also drafted extra clauses for occasional insertion, excluding from its coverage those practicing religious rites "without charge or compensation," as the "best means" of "meeting church objections." For other situations requiring special strategy it prepared a floating clause to meet the opposition of chiropractors, osteopaths, and neuropaths by providing legal exemption for persons "engaging in the administration of massage and similar manual treatment."[37]

The new medical practice laws of the Progressive Era provided no uniform definition of medical practice, but they frequently strengthened the definitions found in olders statutes. Cultists were less successful in evading these laws as the new century advanced. In pleading immunity from such statutes irregular groups increasingly lost in court struggles. The strength of these laws accounts for their effort to secure separate licensing acts and separate examining boards.

LEGISLATING MEDICAL ETHICS

During the Progressive Era the profession both strengthened statutory definitions of medical practice and wrote many of its ethical principles into law. It counterbalanced the growing strains to which these principles were subjected by giving them legal sanction. Seeking genuine professional status for physicians, the AMA renamed its medical "Code" the "Principles of Medical Ethics" in 1903, while constituent societies attempted at the same time to incorporate the ethics into a legal code![38] The profession sought an alliance with the law to remove abuses from within its own ranks that required the exercise of power greater than its own.

States frequently had passed medical laws defining unprofessional conduct before 1900, but as late as 1907 the medical laws of ten states contained no such provisions. A decade later eight of these states had corrected this omission and provided grounds for the revocation of licenses.[39] Furthermore, several states strengthened their laws defining unprofessional practice. The California medical practice law, which named six forms of unprofessional conduct in 1907, listed twelve a decade later, while the number in Iowa's statute rose from four to eleven in the same period.[40]

State laws were much alike in citing certain matters relating to conduct and practice as "unprofessional." These included criminal abortions, proposing to cure incurable diseases, moral turpitude, habitual intemperance, and drug addiction. By 1917 the unprofessional conduct clauses of medical practice laws reflected more faithfully the economic stresses and competitive abuses that disturbed the profession. Only three states had clauses prohibiting physicians from employing "cappers" and "steerers" to acquire patients in 1907, while seven more had such prohibitions a decade later.[41] No state forbade secret fee splitting in 1907, while five states in 1917 had such prohibitions. By 1915, Colorado had added a clause to its medical practice law prohibiting a physician as an employee, partner, or agent of a corporation to treat patients not employed by the enterprise. It became the first state to prohibit the corporate practice of medicine in its practice act.[42]

A NATIONAL LICENSING BOARD

While the regular medical profession usually advanced policies that would place greater restraints on medical practice, it also sought in one area to liberate physicians from the obstructions imposed by a jungle of chaotic medical laws. Diversity of statutes and frequent absence of any reciprocity provisions greatly obstructed the interstate mobility of physicians. The AMA quickly abandoned thought of the establishment of a federal licensing agency, which could not be made both constitutional and effective, or of securing reciprocity through uniform state legislation. By 1902 it favored the creation of a national examining board as proposed by one of its committees. This committee recommended the creation of a board of seven members, including the surgeons-general of the Army, Navy, and Marine-Hospital Service, two elected by the AMA's House of Delegates, one chosen by the American Congress of Physicians and Surgeons, and another by the National Confederation of State Medical Examining and Licensing Boards. Upon the basis of comprehensive examinations it would offer certificates that state examining boards could, but were not under obligation, to accept. The committee believed, however, that as the board acquired a reputation for maintaining high standards its certificates would find wide acceptance.[43]

The proposal for a national board actually ranked low on the AMA's reform agenda. The energy it expended in reorganization and recruitment, reforming medical education, seeking better public health legislation, and combating patent medicine exploitation and other abuses left it too exhausted for many other tasks. Its depleted and imperiled budget did not allow financial support for the work of such a board, nor did organizations representing licensing bodies unite behind this objective. In 1902 the American Confederation of Reciprocating Examining and Licensing Medical Boards broke away from the National Confederation of State Medical Examining and Licensing Boards, hoping to secure reciprocity through licenses based on medical diplomas and sometimes without additional examinations.[44]

Yet hopes for the establishment of a national board survived the disappointments of the decade. Prospects brightened when the Carnegie Foundation for the Advancement of Teaching agreed to subsidize such an operation with an appropriation of $15,000 a year. In 1915, President William L. Rodman, a member of the committee that proposed the board, announced its recent establishment to the House of Delegates at the San Francisco session and plans for the first examination in October at the nation's capital. Within three years the board examined only seventy physicians, but, more important, it had secured recognition in eleven states.[45]

While the regular profession used agencies with no firm legal status (like the national examining board) to serve a special purpose, it secured dominance over areas of health and healing largely through its alliance with the law. This alliance was greatly strengthened in the Progressive Era by a number of decisions rendered by state and federal courts. Upon some medical issues court opinions widely differed; upon some others touching the foundations of the profession's political power courts spoke with remarkable uniformity.[46]

IMPACT OF COURT DECISIONS

Both flourishing and dying sects challenged the constitutionality of the regular profession's dominant position on state health and medical licensing boards, claiming that they could receive no justice from boards largely or totally composed of orthodox physicians. While a few state licensing laws prohibited majority representation of any group, appellate courts generally made no such requirement. When Augustus C. Fowler, an eclectic physician, protested discrimination against eclectics under Louisiana's medical practice act, the state supreme court gave a decision in 1898 (Allopathic State Board of Medical Examiners v. Fowler) that appears to have been followed consistently in the Progressive Era. Its decision stated: "The court knows of no constitutional right given to particular persons, who, entertaining peculiar theories of medicine, group themselves together, and call themselves a special school of medicine under a selected name, to be recognized as and dealt with as such."[47] While the Supreme Court of North Carolina (State v. Biggs) declined to rule in 1903 on whether a form of practice was orthodox or heterodox, the following year the California Supreme Court affirmed *(ex parte Gerino)* that the state had no obligation to give equal board representation to healing sects.[48]

The higher courts generally supported the claims of health and medical examining boards to the power they exercised, and in no area did their decisions have greater impact than in medical education. Repeatedly, court decisions followed the United States Supreme Court's ruling in *Dent* v. *State of West Virginia,* in 1889, holding that the state violated no person's constitutional rights in requiring that every practitioner of medicine within its jurisdiction secure a certificate from the state board of health (or its equivalent) confirming his graduation from a reputable medical college. Thus the fate of medical schools fell largely under the control of boards usually dominated by or fully composed of regular physicians. When the courts ruled early in the twentieth century that boards could judge the reputability of medical colleges by standards that the Association of American Medical Colleges had established, they recognized in effect standards that committees and agencies composed wholly or largely of regular physicians had formulated, interpreted, and applied.[49]

The courts also clarified the rule of administrative agencies in a way that strengthened the position of orthodox medicine by giving little comfort to plaintiffs, shorn of their licenses, who charged that such boards had assumed judicial power illegally and had left them without recourse to due process of law. When Augustus G. Reetz took his case against the Michigan State Board of Registration in Medicine to the United States Supreme Court, contending that the state's medical practice law of 1899 was unconstitutional, Justice David J. Brewer gave the tribunal's opinion in 1902: "The objection that the statute attempts to confer judicial power on the board is not well founded. Many executive officers, even those who are spoken of as purely ministerial officers, act judicially in the determination of facts in the performance of their official duties; and in so doing they do not exercise 'judicial power' as the phrase is commonly used in the organic act in conferring judicial power upon specified courts." He added with appropriate explanations, "Neither is the right of appeal essential to due process of law."[50]

The courts carefully guarded other prerogatives of the boards. Applicants failing licensing examinations had no judicial recourse, said the Idaho Supreme Court:

The courts are open to compel action by the state board of medical examiners when they fail or refuse to act, and to review their authority when they have assumed to exercise powers not conferred; but the board will not review and reexamine matters in which the board is called on to exercise judgment and discretion, and perform *quasi* judicial functions in reference thereto. . . . Courts are neither required nor expected to be experts in therapeutics, gynecology, toxicology, diagnosis, etc., and for them to undertake to examine and grade physicians on such branches would be an unwarranted assumption of jurisdiction.[51]

Sheltered by such important court decisions, state health and medical boards under the control of orthodox medicine wielded enormous power in the Progressive Era. Courts frequently disagreed on whether a particular sect actually practiced medicine, but decisions confirming the broad powers of administrative boards seldom differed.

FIERCENESS OF THE CONFLICT

The fierce conflicts raging between regular and irregular healing groups in state capitals during the Progressive Era have been all but forgotten. One recent writer states incorrectly that not until the compulsory health insurance struggles in the years in and just after World War I did the orthodox profession come to appreciate its political power.[52] Instead, the AMA and its constituent societies tested their strength and displayed their strategy on hundreds of political battlefronts from 1900 to 1910. Perhaps no struggles carried on by other groups were filled with more drama and excitement.

Brief accounts of conflicts in several states illustrate the intensity of the struggle. When the New York Senate Judiciary Committee set hearings in Albany on the osteopathic bill for 29 January 1902, the New York State Medical Society called for its annual meeting to convene at the same time and place. Five hundred regular doctors packed the senate chamber as their spokesmen persuaded the committee to hold up the bill.[53] Four years later the renowned German immigrant and future president of the AMA, Abraham Jacobi, represented the regular profession when osteopaths sought a similar law. He turned tenseness into laughter in the crowded floor and galleries when he exclaimed, "Vat ve vant is to veed them all oudt so they cannot humbug the public for ve know how easy it is to humbug the public." A few months later the *Journal of the American Osteopathic Association* praised the two osteopaths who led the fight: "These are the fellows who stayed up nights; who endured all the horrible, slow, patience-murdering grind, who sweat blood but who saw the thing through."[54]

Tumult reigned in Colorado in 1905 when the regular profession resorted to measures hardly short of violence to secure passage of the new medical practice act. Seymour D. Van Meter, secretary of the State Board of Medical Examiners, rushed to the floor during the voting process, forcing a member into his seat to prevent him from voting against the interests of the profession. For ten days Van Meter had maintained a corps of lobbyists in the house of representatives.[55] In Nebraska in 1901, when the legislature passed an osteopathic bill, the regular profession carried the flight to the governor's office. There the governor listened to a prominent physician debate questions of anatomy with Neil Griffin, who served as his messenger and as custodian of the capitol. Griffin, claiming recently to have been cured by an osteopath, urged the governor to sign the bill. The physician protested in vain as the governor judged Griffin the victor and signed the measure.[56]

In Alabama in 1903 osteopaths confronted the most powerful state medical association in the nation when they sought an independent licensing board. Even before the legislature assembled osteopaths deluged members-elect with literature favorable to their cause. An osteopath from Mobile, Mrs. Ellen Lee Barret Ligon, described even by her opponents as a "beautiful," "fluent," "accomplished," and "cultured" woman, led in the struggle for the measure. The regular profession, long in control of matters of health and medicine, soon knew that it faced perhaps its hardest fight. Obviously alerted by leaders of the state medical association, doctors converged on Montgomery from all parts of the state. Yet the charm, eloquence, and tears of Mrs. Ligon prevailed, and the house passed the measure. When a tie vote followed in the senate only the deciding vote of the lieutenant governor, Russell McWhorter Cunningham, who, fortunately for the embattled doctors, was a regular physician, prevented passage of the bill.[57]

The profession in Kansas in 1912 fought Arthur Capper, who campaigned for the governorship claiming that he had long supported medical cults and patent medicine interests. Most physicians applauded the victory of his Democratic opponent, George H. Hodges, but their rejoicing came too soon. Within a few months he had signed an osteopathic bill and allowed a chiropractic measure to become law without his signature. The editor of the state society's journal lamented that of all the states only Kansas had "legalized" chiropractors. Noting that the chiropractic law required three chiropractors on the board who had practiced within the state for at least two years, he charged that if any chiropractor practiced at all in the state he practiced illegally and was "a criminal in the eyes of the law." Observing that the law also required the appointment of a minister and a schoolteacher, he concluded that they undoubtedly would give the board its only dignity. A year later the editor publicized the votes on previous bills of all candidates for reelection and called for their views on any additional cultist legislation.[58]

The strategy adopted by regular and irregular groups recognized no state boundaries. Sometimes weak irregular groups joined in coalitions to fight orthodox physicians while both irregular and orthodox groups employed extensively the strategy of harassment. The National League of Medical Freedom drew support and sympathy from healing sects who sought to "keep pills out of politics" and feared the growing political power of the AMA as it fought for a national department of public health. The regular profession often harassed irregular groups by insisting on the insertion of meticulous details in laws regulating their practice, while they, in turn, sought legislative restrictions requiring that all prescriptions be prepared in triplicate and explained to patients and that surgeons bear the legal burden of proof in lawsuits that they had performed their work skillfully.[59]

The Progressive Era did not close the dominant profession's conflict with irregular groups, but rather brought victories that largely determined the outcome of the struggle. The strategy it employed in meeting the threat of the emerging sects proved remarkably effective. Through an alliance with the law, largely sanctioned by the courts, it not only repelled forces obstructing the advance of scientific medicine, but secured power important in reaching its economic goals as well. It largely succeeded in depriving irregular groups of credit for pointing out deficiencies in orthodox practice. Its ambivalent strategy in dealing with the dying sects now deserves consideration.

CHAPTER FIVE

THE TALE OF TWO SECTS

The gathering of homeopaths and their well-wishers at Sixteenth and Massachusetts Avenue in the nation's capital late in the afternoon of 21 June 1900 symbolized the hopes of a small, embattled medical organization as it faced the challenges of the new century. Before loyal disciples of Samuel Hahnemann unveiled a statute of their leader, distinguished guests, including President William McKinley, heard tributes to his memory and an ode expressing the profession's confidence in his system:

To us, Sectarians as we ever are
  (As all must be who hold a special creed)
Arose within this country a star
  To guide us in our therapeutic needs.
The storm of opposition touched it not
  The shafts of ridicule pass'd harmless by,
Tradition—dogmas could obscure no jot
  Of its transcendent truth and purity.[1]

HOMEOPATHY: STRENGTH AND WEAKNESS

The homeopaths had some reason for rejoicing. Their movement had reached the United States about 1825 and had survived more than a half-century of struggle following its founder's death in Paris in 1843. By 1900 they claimed nearly thirteen thousand practitioners, and of their twenty medical schools scattered from New York to San Francisco, five had been established in the last decade. In the same decade new state organizations were added in Alabama, South Dakota, and West Virginia, leaving only ten states unorganized, and the number of their publications was raised from twenty to thirty. Furthermore, homeopaths entered the new century with an appreciable measure of

public loyalty varying from the deference of patients who merely preferred the homeopathic approach to the exclusiveness of others whose
only alternative to homeopathic treatment was none at all.[2]

Even as homeopathy assessed its strength and put up its finest front
for public display, it feared threatening and uninviting modern attitudes. As a reform movement it had come far from the era when its
insistence on diminished doses had gained grudging acceptance from
a profession addicted to excessive medication, harsh purgatives, and
bloodletting. It seemed peculiarly unfitted for a medical world that
was becoming specialized and excited by the marvels of preventive
medicine and distrustful of materia medica. The profession in general
saw it as a reactionary body holding out for a discredited therapeutic
principle that associated the cure of disease with the administration of
drugs that produced within the patient the symptoms of the malady
(similia similibus curentur). As a structured medical and metaphysical
system it was even more vulnerable to attack. Founded a half-century
before the advance of the germ theory of disease, it appeared increasingly irrelevant to a profession more scientifically oriented and less
tolerant of dogma.[3]

Late in the nineteenth century homeopaths slowly discovered that
reconciliation of their dogma with scientific medicine was one of their
most urgent tasks. Yet this reconciliation held out before the profession both the hope of survival and the threat of extinction. It could
not reject advances in medical science and survive nor incorporate
them without losing some of its distinctiveness. By 1900 homeopathy
had already lost several of its distinctive features. Many homeopaths
had abandoned inappreciable medication at long intervals for larger
and more frequent doses. No longer did they place reliance, as Hahnemann had, on one drug at a time in treatment or reject specific medication. They now accepted and taught pathology and recognized the
natural causes of disease. Following the lure of surgery some even
strayed after the "orificial" procedures of a notorious Chicago physician, Edwin H. Pratt, whose torturous surgical assaults on the repro-
ductive organs of women with real or imagined gynecological ailments made an advanced science out of mayhem.[4]

As desperate disciples of Hahnemann made scientific adjustments
in their therapeutic system they also recognized that their movement
derived its precarious strength from a wobbly statistical base. They
could find little comfort in a report that associated the strength of

homeopathy with the states having the highest percentages of liter-
acy and that predicted growing popularity for homeopathy with
educational advance.[5] They could cite organizations in thirty-five
states in 1900, but many of these existed in little more than name.
A survey a year later showed the Illinois society with the largest
membership of 690; thirteen state organizations with less than 100
members, four of them less than 25; eight submitting no report at all.
Granting the perhaps exaggerated claim that the movement numbered
nearly 13,000 practitioners in 1900, since only 4,086 homeopathic physicians held membership in state associations, a little less than one-
third of the profession was organized.[6]

BASIC POLICIES

Threats from without and weaknesses within dictated the policies
homeopathic leaders pursued in the new century. Aware of the growing strength of the American Medical Association, they were forced
to expose its monopolistic designs and to resist its efforts to destroy
them. Convinced of the efficacy of their system, they sought to disarm
a hostile scientific world by subjecting their therapeutic principles to
rigid and valid tests. As a final objective, they tried to strengthen and
revitalize their organization as an inevitable move against extinction.

RESISTANCE TO ABSORPTION

Outcries against the efforts of conventional physicians to exterminate the homeopathic system rose to deafening volume early in the
Progressive Era. Behind the two groups lay more than a half-century
of conflict, but homeopaths had discovered that in recent years the
AMA had changed its old strategy of conquest. Inspired by the success
of its timely reorganizational effort, its leaders saw new visions of a
united medical world and a sectless utopia. Their policy against homeopathy involved a greatly renewed emphasis on the strategy of absorption. Substituting cordiality and conciliation for condescension and
contempt, aggressive societies of conventional physicians sought to
lure and embrace discouraged and unsuspecting homeopaths. For
others more resistant to this approach the AMA had a firmer and more
compelling strategy. Through a tightening alliance with the federal
and state governments it hoped to convince outnumbered homeopaths
of overwhelming pressures that could be employed to destroy their
system.[7]

Even before 1900, suspicious homeopaths had warned of modera-
tion in the AMA's hostility which concealed, they believed, its ultimate objective of destroying their movement "by prehension, mastica-
tion, deglutition, digestion and assimiliation."[8] Yet not until examples
mounted after the new century began did they offer convincing evidence of a plot and identify the plotters. To George H. Simmons,
secretary of the AMA, editor of its *Journal* (and a former homeopath),
and to Charles A. L. Reed of Cincinnati, chairman of the AMA's Committee on Medical Legislation, they ascribed responsibility for its
bold strategy. After a decade of acquaintance with Simmons's alleged
intrigues, which included no critical reference to homeopathy in the
Journal, a Los Angeles practitioner summed up homeopathic opinion
in charging that the editor was a "scheming politician" trying to wreck
their system. Henry E. Beebe, a prominent homeopath of Sidney,
Ohio, publicized his own experiences as a victim of the AMA's absorption plan first employed at Dayton. Upon Reed's insistence, Beebe
agreed to attend a dinner at which the Cincinnati physician presented
a paper and more than complied with his promise by bringing along
several homeopathic associates. Though all vowed in advance that they
would not join Reed's organization, at the registration desk they were
called upon to pay one dollar: fifty cents for the dinner and fifty cents
for membership. Before the hour had passed the bewildered men
found themselves members of a regular association from which they
succeeded in extricating themselves three weeks later.[9]

Homeopathic leaders found more than isolated instances to support
their charges of seduction. The AMA had established ample grounds
for its own indictment when it promoted a reorganizational plan that
during and after 1903 allowed local societies, which long had shunned
homeopathic contacts, to admit any legally registered and reputable
physician to membership who was not supporting an exclusive system,
practicing by its principles, or claiming to do so. Since homeopaths
made no pretense to exclusiveness they found the energies of many
local organizations directed toward their absorption. The Massachusetts Medical Society admittedly had their inclusion in mind when it
lowered its barriers in 1906 to include physicians claiming adherence
to no exclusive system.[10] As early as 1904, a prominent leader of the
AMA had urged the acceptance of homeopaths without even requiring detachment from their own organizations, and a year later William
Osler unwittingly confirmed their fears when in his farewell address

to regular physicians (who assembled to bestow upon him due honor before he began his distinguished career at Oxford) he included reconciliation with homeopathy as one of the profession's three most urgent needs. Evidence also indicated that homeopathic leaders had acted none too soon in attempting to hold their threatened ranks against desertion. A Texas fugitive from the movement reported in 1906 that although most homeopaths retained faith in their therapeutic principles, 90 percent would readily abandon their distinctive designation.[11]

When the Philadelphia County Medical Society resolved in 1907 to admit any legally qualified physician who agreed "not to accept any sectarian designation or base his practice on any exclusive dogma or system," a homeopathic editor quickly sensed the gravity of the threat. Ruling out any idea that local regular physicians had repented of repeated acts of intolerance and persecution, he assigned three reasons for their strategy. They hoped to profit financially, he believed, from professional consultation with homeopaths. But he charged that primarily they sought an alliance to strengthen their position in the struggle for a new medical practice act, and that after the passage of such a law they planned to exterminate the movement by absorption when it could no longer serve a political end.[12]

Faithful homeopaths confessed to bewilderment as the beguiling strategy of the AMA spread disaffection within their ranks. Their dream of peaceful coexistence within the community of healing began to vanish before the dominant profession's intrigue and subversion. For them the AMA offered no more than an ultimatum to surrender, which they must meet with firmness and defiance. Beebe set forth what may be regarded as the homeopathic manifesto when he declared that amalgamation inevitably would come, but only when the orthodox profession accepted homeopathic principles.[13]

SCIENTIFIC RIVALRY

Well aware that the subtle strategy of the AMA could not be dismissed simply with words of warning, homeopathic leaders attempted to draw the association into conflict on its apparently most vulnerable front. They proposed to carry the fight into the sector of science and to establish the superiority of their therapeutic system by reliable and thorough tests. In this area of combat they were confident of victory and eager to meet what they looked upon as an arrogant and insulting foe. For years they had heard prominent regular physicians confess to the worthlessness of nearly all of the drugs used in orthodox practice but assail the homeopathic system as built on "absurd foundations," "absolutely and fundamentally unscientific," and, like the American Indian, "an anachronism" in a progressive age. Fully convinced that objective research and experimentation on drug action would confirm the "law of similars," defenders of homeopathy hoped to establish their claim over an area from which defenseless conventional practitioners converted to therapeutic nihilism had fled.[14]

In 1908 the American Institute of Homeopathy appointed a committee to appeal to the AMA for a "joint investigation of the scientific merits of the method of drug selection," which the formula "Similia Similibus Curentur" expressed. This appeal brought no favorable response and never received the attention of more than a few members of the House of Delegates. The AMA already had placed ethical drugs under some measure of surveillance through its newly created Council on Pharmacy and Chemistry and made no effort to move into the much larger area of actually searching out effective remedies.[15]

Repelled by the AMA, the American Institute of Homeopathy undertook its own investigation, organizing the American Association of Clinical Research for this purpose in October 1909. The institute expected this body to develop an "absolutely conclusive clinical method" for proving the principles and facts of medicine "to the absolute satisfaction of an impossible rejection of any of the various factions of medicine, old and new, sectarian and non-sectarian."[16] Less than a year later it reported that the Massachusetts Homeopathic Hospital had agreed to conduct research through the senior staff of the medical board and that two other hospitals in Louisville and St. Louis contemplated similar work. Other institutions soon announced their research intentions. In Chicago, the Hering Medical College planned the construction of the "Constantine Hering Laboratory" for investigations in therapeutics and pharmacodynamics, and the Hahnemann Medical College proposed an enlargement of its laboratories. The New York Homeopathic Medical College constructed a new laboratory for bacteriological and pathological research, and in California the Hahnemannian College of the Pacific made similar improvements. Placing greater reliance on clinical research than on laboratory investigation, homeopaths believed that the work conducted by their institutions would far surpass in importance that of the Council of Pharmacy and Chemistry of the AMA.[17]

Ever hoping for a scientific confrontation with conventional medicine, the American Institute of Homeopathy issued another challenge to the AMA a half-decade after it rejected the first. Offering to subject the law of similars to any scientific test, it proposed a joint investigation under the auspices of such research centers as the McCormack Institute of Chicago or the Rockefeller Institute of New York. It also sought the AMA's cooperation by stressing the importance of testing drugs common to both systems. Furthermore, by notifying the editors of twenty regular, eleven homeopathic, and two eclectic journals of its appeal, the institute added considerable pressure to its persuasion.[18]

When the AMA responded somewhat favorably to the institute's proposal, the homeopathic leadership was surprised that its persistence had been rewarded. It ascribed credit to Abraham Jacobi, the renowned pediatrician and president of the AMA, for successfully pressing the matter upon the association's governing body. Yet Jacobi's move came at a most appropriate time. Within the AMA's own membership scattered protests that therapeutic research had been neglected jarred organizational apathy and the Pharmacopoeial Convention of 1910 had served as an embarrassing decennial reminder of the uncertainty and ignorance surrounding drug administration and action.[19] A recent survey of drugs most frequently employed by physicians had revealed the embarrassing fact that cactus, declared "utterly worthless" as a remedy by the Council on Pharmacy and Chemistry of the AMA, led the entire list. Voices abroad even joined the outcry, and while negotiations with homeopaths were still under way the famous British heart specialist, James MacKenzie, announced in January 1914 that "not one single drug has been carefully studied so as to understand its full effect on the human system."[20]

The courses of the two organizations converged briefly at the threshold of science. In the spring of 1914 the rival bodies sought the services of three independent laboratories to conduct their investigations. Two of these showed only enough interest to respond unfavorably and the third did not reply. On 3 July as the tensions of Europe sizzled toward the explosion of World War I, the AMA called upon the institute to offer some other practical method of investigation. Subsequent negotiations are somewhat obscure, but the two organizations could bring no research program into being. No longer did Jacobi remain as president of the AMA to press for joint investigations, and the shock of World War I raised many diverting issues. Even the uni-

lateral commercial drug testing of the AMA's Council on Pharmacy
and Chemistry seemed imperiled the next year when the council, dis-
mayed by what it thought were the meager accomplishments of a
decade, hinted at the propriety of its own dissolution.[21]

Homeopathic leadership did not entirely rest its case for survival
upon warning its scattered followers of the AMA's designs or in seeking scientific vindication. The growing threat of the AMA early in the
second decade of the century brought forth belated but bolder strategy. Ever convinced that the newly issued Carnegie Foundation report
on medical education and the newly proposed national health department bill represented sinister attempts by the AMA to exterminate
homeopathic colleges and to gain enormous political leverage, the
institute rallied its strength for a crucial struggle.[22] It sought to restore
unity and tolerance within its ranks and to extend its membership by
a nationwide recruitment crusade.

APPEAL FOR TOLERANCE

The institute employed the threat of the AMA to achieve unity, but
also appealed to detached homeopaths by confronting issues that
divided the group with the widest margin of tolerance. In 1912 a
prominent leader of the institute, Royal S. Copeland, drew up a
homeopathic credo that called for acceptance of the law of similars
as a working hypothesis but stressed the great latitude of opinion the
principle allowed. He emphasized the "virtue of the small dose," but
contended that the "exact size and form" should be matters of individual selection. He raised no objection to the use of adjuvants and pal-
liatives, and while stressing the sufficiency of the "perfectly selected
homeopathic remedy," he recognized the usefulness of mechanical and
chemical therapy. Finally, he reminded homeopaths of one of their
cherished mottoes that fittingly expressed their tolerance:

> In essentials, harmony;
> In non-essentials, liberty;
> In all, charity.[23]

RECRUITMENT CRUSADE

The institute did not rely only on a generous display of charity and
tolerance to strengthen the movement but searched for ways to extend
the organization into the homeopathic hinterlands. As early as 1907,

at the annual session of the institute, Hugo R. Arndt of Cleveland urged that a national campaign of promotion be begun citing as a model the successful expansion work of the AMA. At the same session a Chicago homeopath emphasized the urgency of action when he warned the institute that in some states homeopathy was fighting to retain its position, in many it was fighting for existence, and in others it was not fighting at all. Homeopathic leadership made its first response to this warning when it established the *Journal of the American Institute of Homeopathy* on 1 January 1909, hoping to attract detached members of the profession.[24]

Not relying exclusively on the printed word, the institute took its boldest step in 1910 when it selected a field secretary, and Arndt, who proposed the action three years before, accepted the appointment. Arndt hoped both to awaken the profession and to appeal to the public. He soon discovered that the sweep of therapeutic nihilism had not destroyed public confidence in the system and that localities desiring homeopaths far exceeded the supply. Attempting to publicize the movement, he prepared two leaflets designed for physicians to use in explaining homeopathy to patients and entitled *What Homeopathy Is* and *What Homeopathy Is Not*. Other homeopaths endorsed Arndt's effort to reach the people for professional vindication. Contending that the public knew its needs in medicine just as in politics and religion, Pinkerton Crutcher of Kansas City gladly agreed to turn over the fate of the system to this "Great Court of Final Appeal."[25]

In November 1910, Arndt reported on his first recruitment mission which extended over more than five weeks, moving eastward from the Pacific Coast. Visiting Spokane, Denver, Chicago, Pittsburgh, Philadelphia, and several other cities, he found much room for hope. Convinced that sustained organizational effort would revive the movement, he announced that "homeopathy quiescent will soon become homeopathy militant, and homeopathy militant will eventually become homeopathy triumphant." Six months later he reported that he had visited homeopathic societies in twenty-one states and made from one to seven addresses in each state. Furthermore, he had visited most of the homeopathic colleges, counseling and encouraging students.[26]

Late in 1911, Arndt announced that the South would be the scene of his next major drive. Recognizing that feeble southern societies needed "new men to bring new life," he confessed that his greatest expectation was to help "discouraged and half beaten forces" hold

their own ground. But after working in much of the South he gave up
even this modest hope. Early in 1912 he found southern homeopaths
so scattered that cooperation was more difficult among them than
among their brethren in the Far West.[27]

When the institute held its annual session in July, Arndt reported
on the travels of a strenuous year. He had carried his enlistment work
into seventeen states and had visited eight others. In only nine states
of the nation had he failed to carry his recruitment campaign. Although his report was fairly encouraging, this session held little more
than disappointment for him. The trustees announced that the virtual
exhaustion of funds prevented renewal of his contract beyond its expir-
ation date in late September and declared that they would decide on
a future recruitment policy at a meeting in December. Yet their
acceptance of a proposal for the solicitation of two dollars a year for
five years from all homeopaths for continuing this work offered some
hope.[28] Although the trustees announced at the December meeting
that they would extend the contract to at least the middle of the following year, an unexpected incident quickly brought this form of
organizational effort to an end. Arndt, upon whom most of the responsibility for promotional work depended, died on 2 January 1913, and
the future of the program remained in doubt.[29]

The homeopathic Council on Medical Education soon took up the
burden that Arndt had borne and laid out a broader program of work.
It announced plans to issue a small publication, the *News Letter*, that
first appeared in January 1914. It proposed a lectureship program to
reach the public and a plan of instruction for college students who
promised to follow a homeopathic career. It pledged protection to the
profession against hostile legislation appearing at state and national
capitals and greater cooperation within the profession. Finally, it
promised to employ an organizer as a successor to Arndt although it
never did.[30]

HOMEOPATHIC DECLINE

Despite exertions of the institute after the death of Arndt, evidence
mounted that the movement was declining. Shortly before his death
prominent homeopaths expressed fears about the fate of their system.
Willis A. Dewey found that some of the forces retarding the movement included collaboration with the "old school," use of textbooks
of the regular profession in homeopathic colleges, and lack of coopera-

tion and organization. William H. Van den Burg gave as the most important reasons for decline the unpopularity of drug therapy; growing stress on surgery; and greater recourse to hygienic, dietary, and climatic treatment. But to this he added the advance in bacteriology and the growth of serum and vaccine therapy. Furthermore, he and another homeopath, Rudolph F. Rabe, found that aversion within their ranks to the restrictive principles of sectarian systems had weakened the movement.[31]

Seeking almost any formula for survival, homeopathic leadership appealed to another imperiled sect. In June 1915 the president of the institute addressed the annual session of the National Eclectic Med ical Association in San Francisco, stressing the similarities between the groups and urging a merger of the movements. Much of the leadership within the dying sects favored the union, but the proposal raised opposition among those who chose to decline separately. Rather pathetically the *Homeopathic Recorder* confessed some fourteen months later that "the older homeopaths are dying off, and their places are not being filled," attributing the loss to the greater attraction of the trades and of professions other than medicine.[32]

At the end of the Progressive Era a few homeopaths could recall the exciting day in 1900 when they gathered in Washington to publicize and revive their movement. In the intervening years they saw instead the rapid decline of their system. Only skeleton organizations remained in many states, and none at all in others. Of their twenty medical schools in 1900, eleven had fallen before the AMA's movement for educational reform. The fate of their system lay in the future of their colleges. On 3 March 1917, Royal S. Copeland, dean of the New York Medical College and Flower Hospital, labeled the colleges "sanctuaries" of the faith and urged a "Pentecostal Revival." Designating 19 October as a "Rally Day or Pentecost," he called on homeopaths who had not outlived their alma maters to come back to strengthen and share their faith.[33]

The desperate exertions of homeopathy at the end of the Progressive Era rate as little more than the futile responses of an enfeebled sect to the near certainty of virtual extinction. Five years later all but two of its schools had closed, and while these institutions retained a commitment to the system beyond the middle of the century, their loyalties became increasingly ineffectual and remote.[34] The homeopathic movement brought to the new era too little strength, while science imposed too many demands. Nor could homeopathy deal successfully with the ambivalent strategy of the regular profession. As orthodox leaders lured many practitioners, they deprived homeopathic colleges of access to great reservoirs of Carnegie and Rockefeller wealth, which saved and strengthened many colleges of their own. The great burden of medical education gradually fell largely on the public, but by 1917 the regular profession, practically dictating the use of public wealth, was firmly in control.

ECLECTIC MOVEMENT: ITS SURVIVAL

As homeopathy struggled almost futilely against the hostile forces of the new century the strivings of the eclectic movement followed much the same course. Smaller than the homeopathic sect and never numbering more than nine thousand physicians, eclectics matched the larger group primarily in their determination to survive. More than a half-century lay behind the movement that found its origin in a faction nurtured on the medical ideas of Worcester Beach, who established his own medical school in Cincinnati in 1842.[35] Eclectics had survived the ravages of sectarian warfare and the advance of preventive medicine that had threatened their movement with extinction. Facing the new century, they saw even greater dangers as the growing popularity of therapeutic nihilism boded ill for a system that justified its existence on the efficiency of its drug therapy.

No reliable statistics reveal the actual size of the eclectic sect in 1900, but information gathered seven years later adequately portrays the strength of the movement in the first decade. A careful study found eclectics practicing in every state, but in fourteen they numbered no more than twenty-five, and in five others less than fifty. In thirteen states the movement had no state organizations, and in fifteen no members in the National Eclectic Medical Association. Only in California, Illinois, Indiana, Missouri, New York, and Ohio did eclectic practitioners exceed 400, and of a total of 7,464 practicing eclectics, only 2,345 held state society membership, and only 508 belonged to the national body.[36]

The National Eclectic Medical Association found in the diminishing outflow of eight eclectic medical schools its chance to replenish the reserves of a movement already ominously weakened by apathy and erosion. Struggling eclectic medical schools extended from coast to coast, but the Eclectic Medical Institute of Cincinnati held greatest promise of endurance. Relying on the great library of two brothers, John Uri Lloyd and Curtis Gates Lloyd, whose acquisitions of literature on botany, pharmacy, and materia medica surpassed any in the world, the Cincinnati school had an advantage over all others. Yet even this school, which graduated only 174 students in the first half-decade of the twentieth century, was a feeble bulwark against forces endangering the movement.[37]

ECLECTIC HOPES

Eclectics based their hopes of survival on the alleged superiority of their remedies. One observed that "as a school we do not profess to be superior in all departments of medicine, but in the domain of medical treatment we do profess to stand supreme." The editor of the *Eclectic Medical Journal* distinguished eclectic physicians from all others by "their thorough knowledge of American-plant medicines and the administration of a remedy for certain definite symptoms of disease expressions instead of . . . diagnosing a disease and then prescribing for the name." Contending that the therapeutic action of drugs could not be tested experimentally by their poisonous effects on animals, another prominent eclectic, Albert F. Stephens, contrasted the "*harsh, poisonous, destructive* treatment" of other systems with the "kindly, humane, nonpoisonous, curative treatment of eclecticism."[38]

Most eclectics readily accepted the sectarian label. In 1903, John Uri Lloyd contended that sects in medicine, as well as in religion, served to "strengthen," "broaden," and "deepen" the accomplishments of both. Stephens also defended sectarianism, but insisted that it be of a congenial type, while another eclectic described the system as "nothing more or less than a broad liberality untrammeled by codes or prejudices" and liberal enough to accept all medical truth.[39] Naturally, eclectics fought all legislative proposals that favored one medical group over another. They still adhered to the view of John King, a pioneer in the movement, who believed that true eclecticism and Americanism had to confer on all medical sects the same freedom that it readily granted to bakers and grocers.[40]

RESISTING ABSORPTION

Eclectic leaders, long inured to the bitterness of medical-group conflict, quickly discovered their principal adversary in the Progressive Era. As the American Medical Association brought its nationwide reorganizational effort toward completion and pressed more subtly its campaign of absorption, alarmed eclectics knew that their movement faced its gravest threat. Perceiving the danger even more readily than did homeopaths, they moved just as vigorously to meet the challenge.

One eclectic editor offered proof that regular societies had employed the most deceptive strategy in attempting to absorb the movement by not requiring the abandonment of either sectarian practice or designation in granting membership. He cited no less an authority than Charles A. L. Reed, of the AMA's Committee on Medical Legislation, who maintained that since 1901 all "arbitrary rules and absurd barriers" to union had been removed.[41] Confirming this view, the editor of the *Eclectic Medical Journal* cited the case of Peter D. Bixel of Pandora, Ohio, classified by the AMA as one of its members, who repeatedly had rejected overtures from the local regular society though the solicitation for membership required no concessions. He also cited the remarks of the editor of the *Virginia Semi-Monthly*, an orthodox publication, who, opposing the AMA's strategy, charged that conventional societies in the haste of reorganization had fallen into the "trap" of promoting absorption.[42]

Eclectic leaders warned that members straying into regular folds later would be forced to abandon sectarian designation however much regular societies might conceal their demand. One editor insisted that no eclectic, however regular in "habits and bowels" and in his "emissions, omissions and commissions," could escape the "regular" appellation in an orthodox brotherhood.[43] A California physician warned eclectics who were tempted by the strategy of absorption of the man in the familiar fable who "in driving his ass to market tried to please everybody, pleased nobody, and lost his ass in the bargain." Without indicating how many permanent losses eclecticism had suffered, in 1909, John K. Scudder informed the unwary of the disillusionment defectors experienced before returning to the security of the fold.[44]

Many eclectics shared with homeopaths a growing suspicion of the AMA's gestures of friendship. Why, asked Stephens in 1907, had the Texas and New York legislatures destroyed their systems of three licensing boards to create only one, and why had the state board of Missouri so recently displayed hostility toward sectarian medical schools? The regular profession hoped, he contended, to control legislatures, to dictate appointments to administrative medical posts, and to destroy most medical schools that had no university affiliations.

Three years later eclectics charged that the AMA's designs had broadened into a national strategy. The National Eclectic Medical Association denounced the Owen national health department bill as an effort by the AMA to employ federal power against them.[45]

THERAPEUTIC CONTROVERSY

Not only did eclectics oppose the seductive strategy of the AMA and its alleged drive for political dominance; they also carried on a continuous dispute over therapeutic issues that long had raised dissension. An era that produced the greatest triumphs in preventive medicine only deepened the conflict as regular physicians increasingly despaired of the efficacy of drug remedies. Not yet convinced of the virtues of vaccine and serum therapy, many eclectics held that the influence of the AMA largely accounted for the diminishing emphasis on drug treatment. Yet, while attacking the AMA for its neglect of materia medica, they resented its acceptance of new synthetic drugs that were largely of German origin to the exclusion of botanical preparations.[46]

The controversy took its bitterest turn when enraged eclectics found editors of regular journals pirating remedies of the sect and extolling their virtues as new discoveries. In March 1900, W. C. Cooper, coeditor of the *Eclectic Medical Gleaner,* reported such an instance and branded an editor as "either an ignoramous or a d——d whelp." A decade later Rolla L. Thomas of the Cincinnati eclectic school exposed the alleged subtlety of the AMA in occasionally acquiring eclectic remedies. He contended that the Council on Pharmacy and Chemistry would accept them only when they had filtered in from Europe and when it could escape embarrassment by attributing their discovery to a foreign source.[47]

RECRUITMENT EFFORT

Sporadic journalistic attacks over matters of ethics and therapeutics portrayed the resentment within eclectic ranks rather than a revival of the system. Slowly eclectic leaders decided that nothing less than a vigorous promotional effort directed by the national organization could revive the movement. By February 1908 the national association had appointed a Committee on Organization that consisted of one physician in each of thirty-two states, with separate recruiters for Cincinnati and Chicago. Although the national body established the general organizational plan, the Ohio association worked out a more complex pattern. In addition to a state organizer, its president announced that he would follow the plan of the regular profession by dividing the state into ten districts with an official organizer in each.[48]

In June 1909 the annual session of the association unanimously voted to discard the *Transactions* and to establish a quarterly that would assist the organization in its recruitment drive. In September the first issue of the *National Eclectic Medical Association Quarterly* appeared, pledging to place the association in closer contact with the work of state societies and their auxiliaries. It made no effort to conceal dangers facing the movement, indicating that the greatest was the AMA's attempt to destroy eclectic medical colleges.[49]

Favorable response within the profession to the recruitment program convinced skeptical eclectic leaders of the propriety of their effort. Application forms circulated through state secretaries and through the *Quarterly* brought hundreds of membership requests. At the annual session of 1909, the association admitted more than 400 new members, and in September 1910 the national secretary reported that approximately 600 applicants had been granted membership since the midyear session. These gains appeared all the more impressive compared to the total membership of only 442 in 1900.[50]

COLLAPSING MOVEMENT

Yet the feverish promotional enthusiasm that reached its crest early in the second decade quickly began to subside. The national organization showed no capacity to sustain an effective recruitment program, nor could it protect the group from the alienating influence of regular physicians though it expelled the Illinois society for succumbing to their seduction. It could give little assistance to eclectic colleges or persuade many youths to take up careers in eclectic medicine.[51]

In 1913, William N. Mundy, chairman of the Committee on Organization, laid bare to the association the general status of the organizational movement. To each unorganized eclectic practitioner in the nation he recently had addressed a personal appeal that had brought no impressive response. While commending the work of state recruiters in California, New York, Illinois, Missouri, and Georgia, he found that in some states even the organizers had not joined the national association, and he listed many states with very few eclectic practitioners. He called for the maintenance of societies even in these states, but recommended that physicians in them follow the example of the South Dakota society and hold joint meetings with homeopaths. William P. Best, the recording secretary, offered the association an equally discouraging report. He considered the widespread membership delinquency that reached as high as 67 percent in Nebraska and 73 percent in Illinois adequate evidence of "startling inefficiency, lack of interest or total loss."[52]

Weakened by indifference and desertion, the eclectic movement faced still other dangers. Against its struggling schools the American Medical Association had launched a fierce attack supported by Carnegie and Rockefeller wealth. Two of the eight eclectic schools had perished before the first decade ended, and four others had collapsed by 1915, when an eclectic editor spoke of the jeopardy in which the "great moneyed interests" had placed the movement. Still another, the Georgia College of Eclectic Medicine and Surgery, that traced its roots to the rubble of war-wrecked Atlanta, fell a year later, leaving only the Cincinnati school when the Progressive Era closed.[53]

Late in 1916 the eclectic Committee on Organization complained to the annual session of the virtual collapse of the recruitment program while the president of the association ritualistically announced high hopes for the movement. Yet even a persistent enlistment effort probably would have done little more than retard decline. A year earlier an eclectic editor had observed and explained the trend. He referred to the success of the AMA's strategy of seduction in permanently alienating some practitioners. He spoke of the spread of therapeutic nihilism that had brought eclectic drug theory into disrepute and of the contributions serums and vaccines had made to preventive medicine. He claimed that the appeal of mechanotherapy had carried wayward eclectics even into chiropractic and osteopathic ranks. In opposing an effort to reverse the trend through a merger with homeopathy, but in offering no plan for revival, he appeared to consign the movement to inevitable extinction.[54]

CHAPTER SIX

PHYSICIANS AND PUBLIC HEALTH REFORM

P The regular medical profession matched its triumphs over competing medical groups in the Progressive Era with substantial victories in areas of public health. At a time when much of the profession had lost confidence in the efficacy of curative medicine, advances in immunology tended to shake further the profession's confidence in its own usefulness. Yet as physicians moved through their societies to take over partial leadership of the public health crusade and struggled to acquaint the public with the sources and prevention of diseases, they not only performed much of their greatest service but gained in public esteem as well. The challenge of the public health movement had still another effect on the profession. When physicians lost nearly 40 percent of their case load with the advance of the revolution in preventive medicine in the quarter-century before 1912, they struggled all the more desperately to prevent encroachments upon their practice from proprietary medical houses and healing sects.[1]

SPECTRUM OF REFORM

Few matters falling into the range of conventional public health legislation lay beyond the profession's interest in the Progressive Era. Such problems as the exploitation of child labor and women workers, hazards to life and health in industrial production, slum congestion, and oppression of blacks raised little interest within the profession when many other organized groups and the public generally supported these abuses or made no effort to prevent them. But on many fronts to which the profession brought expertise and familiarity, it assisted immeasurably in reversing growing threats to health and in advancing the revolution in preventive medicine. Early in 1914, Frederick R. Green, secretary of the AMA's Council on Health and Public Instruction, outlined the profession's minimum goals, most of which it had already achieved. His list included adequate medical practice laws and vital statistics legislation, basic public health laws, the establishment of local health units, and the coordination of their activities with the work of state boards of health. He added food and drugs laws and legislation providing for safer water supplies and proper sewage disposal and for sanitary surveys of the states. Legislation providing means for the reduction of industrial diseases, for milk inspection, and for medical inspection of public schools completed his list.[2] These proposed minimum standards suggested that the profession also had comprehensive goals and other special interests. The former included instruction of the entire nation on matters of public health, while the latter included such pervasive problems as the prevention of infant blindness (opthalmia neonatorum) and puerperal fever.

VARIATIONS OF RESPONSE

A survey of the public health work of the profession requires some reservations. By no means did all medical societies join the struggle for reform, and some gave no more than passive support to the public health movement. Frequently, while fighting for public health measures, they attempted to work out clear zones between public health and private practice and to prevent encroachments on the latter. Few within the profession recognized that the growing complexities of the economic order sorely challenged the adequacy of conventional methods for the administration and payment of medical care. Some state societies had no official organs to alert and mobilize physicians, and others found that their journals reached only a part of their membership and that much of this group read their columns only irregularly. Furthermore, the medical profession often allowed other organizations to take over leadership in public health crusades and rarely could claim full credit for reforms. But even these reservations must not detract from the profession's work and its immeasurable accomplishments in areas of public health. Advancing causes that often adversely affected their economic interests, physicians overcame much of the public's apathy toward public health matters in less than two decades.

THE CASE OF KANSAS

No state association made greater contributions to public health reform than did the society in Kansas, and no state accomplished more.

Although the gains in Kansas are atypical, they show how a distinguished secretary of the state board of health, Samuel J. Crumbine, drew state agencies, medical societies, and enlightened organizations of laymen into an alliance that left a record of achievement envied by medical leaders throughout the nation. In January 1913 the *Journal of the Kansas Medical Society* listed twenty-one public health reforms in which Kansas took the lead, yet this list failed fully to portray the record as it omitted the establishment of the board of health in 1885 and the passage of two medical practice laws for which Kansas could claim no priority. Furthermore, the list represented gains achieved not as much by legislation as by administrative implementation, all of which seem to have occurred after 1904 when Crumbine's public service began.[3]

Kansas ranked as the first state to establish a summer school to provide physicians and health officials with better training for public health work and to place officials administering the food and drugs legislation under civil service. It was the first state to provide a portable emergency hypochlorite plant for purifying city water in typhoid epidemics and the first to outlaw the public drinking cup and roller towel on public carriers. Kansas led all other states in establishing a quarterly inspection of packing house employees to detect contagious diseases, introduced the national campaign to "swat the fly," and educational films for public health demonstrations, and conducted the first social study of vital statistics. While the state health board made these advances with the cooperation of physicians, it also secured their aid in combating ophthalmia neonatorum and in securing data on tuberculosis and cancer. In 1915 the medical profession and the board of health saw much of their struggle against tuberculosis bear fruit when the state opened its first sanitarium at Norton.[4]

STATE BOARDS OF HEALTH

Medical associations well knew that the success of their public health campaigns would depend in large measure on the power of state boards of health. When Arizona, Georgia, and Oregon established boards in 1902, leaving only Idaho with no such agency, medical societies turned increasingly to the task of strengthening them. State health boards, usually meagerly financed, spread their work thinly over many areas. In 1905 the *Texas State Journal of Medicine* carried an article surveying board functions in five states, noting that they fell in ten principal areas. Four of these included control over quarantine, stream pollution, communicable diseases, and "health nuisances." The boards also supervised vaccination, compilation of vital statistics, and food and drugs legislation. The other areas included responsibility for the treatment of the insane, regulation of the transportation of dead bodies, and coordination of the health work of local agencies.[5] The profession generally attached greatest importance to the latter function, believing that the creation of additional local health boards and the coordination of their work with state health agencies would ensure the success of most public health reforms. Furthermore, it did not restrict itself to objectives that got high priority from health boards and sometimes pioneered along paths of its own.

GREAT WHITE PLAGUE ATTACKED

Against the great white plague (tuberculosis) that defied all advances in immunology, physicians made some of their most impressive contributions in the Progressive Era. Because they often encountered the ravages wrought by the disease they read with no surprise statistics provided by the *Illinois Medical Journal* for the year 1904, showing that deaths from tuberculosis in the state exceeded deaths from eight other major diseases combined. Physicians had supported the few organizations struggling against the menace before the National Association for the Study and Prevention of Tuberculosis was created in 1904, and they helped raise the total number of these groups to 1,228 nine years later.[6] Early in the new century several associations appointed committees to draft petitions to legislatures urging the establishment of sanitariums, and spokesmen for state societies addressed legislatures on ways to control the disease. Much of their work, when combined with comparable efforts of other organizations, was remarkably effective. Only Massachusetts and New York had established state sanitariums by 1901, and only a few private sanitariums existed. By 1908 eighteen states had provided homes for tubercular patients, and by 1913 the number of public and private hospitals and sanitariums devoted to the treatment of the disease reached 527, not including 395 dispensaries.[7]

When Maryland completed construction of one of the nation's finest sanitariums in 1908, the *Maryland Medical Journal* rejoiced and asked the profession to prove that the expenditure was justified. But this project only augmented physicians' efforts to combat tuberculosis under earlier laws. In 1904 the legislature passed a measure requiring compulsory registration of tubercular cases and another that established what became known as the "Maryland System." This plan, quickly adopted in several other states, required disinfection of private homes in which tubercular patients had died. It established stations at which prophylactic supplies could be secured at state expense, upon requisition of physicians, and prescribed a small remuneration for their compliance with the act.[8] Other decentralized forms of tubercular patient care appeared when several states adopted laws granting county supervisors power to establish local public hospitals. By 1911 six states adopted laws with this provision, helping to implement the goals of much of the profession. But even this system fell short of the proposals of some physicians. When President William E. McVey addressed a meeting of the Kansas Medical Society on the advantages of cottage treatment over all others, the organization submitted his plan to the legislature, but it showed no interest.[9]

The profession did not rely on institutional confinement or disinfection procedures to defeat the tuberculosis scourge and laid its principal hopes on a campaign of national education. Only the public, it believed, when properly informed of the hazards of the disease and methods of prevention, could stop its spread. In 1910, John B. Hawes II told the Massachusetts Medical Society that education of the public rated with the isolation of advanced cases of consumption as the most important aspects of the struggle. Yet earlier McVey lamented that the government had spent much money to instruct the public on fattening hogs, raising cattle, and caring for milk cows, "but not one dollar to protect our children from the ravages of this insidious, slow, far-reaching, terribly prevalent, and fearfully fatal disease."[10] During this era medical societies did much to overcome government's default at both the state and federal levels.

The crusade of medical societies took several forms. Many societies established committees to investigate the subject and supported two international conferences on tuberculosis, one in Baltimore in 1904 and another at the nation's capital four years later. The Baltimore conference provided much of the inspiration for the profession's efforts to establish branches of the National Association for the Study and Prevention of Tuberculosis after its creation in 1904, and through these branches, composed of physicians and laymen, to conduct statewide crusades. Some societies moved slowly to establish branches and very likely several never did, but all state organizations seem to have contributed to the movement.[11]

The Pennsylvania society established a speakers' panel, for the instruction of physicians and laymen alike, and called on medical societies to discuss the matter. When the Georgia association established a branch of the national association it urged the presentation of lectures in public schools. In 1910 the Massachusetts society helped to secure a small legislative appropriation for the preparation of school exhibits on tuberculosis, and throughout this era most journals devoted considerable attention to the problem.[12] In 1915 the Michigan society announced that the legislature had appropriated $100,000 for a survey of tuberculosis in the state. It set aside a Tuberculosis Day and urged physicians to donate their services in examining individuals who sought their aid. The following year the society set 10 August as Tuberculosis Day on which physicians examined 442 patients and diagnosed 139 as tubercular. The society in Kansas, like many more, established a branch of the national association as well as its own Committee on Tuberculosis Prevention. But, unlike others, it could combine its work with the campaign waged by the nation's most influential state board of health.[13] Countless physicians worked tirelessly in the crusade rendering their services through innumerable agencies or individual action. For example, Frank Billings, an outstanding Chicago medical educator, who served twice as president of the AMA, served also as president of the state Board of Charities which turned its attention to the problem, and in 1908, William R. M. Kellogg, a Seattle physician, established a journal devoted to discussions of the disease.[14]

MEDICAL INSPECTION OF SCHOOLS

The medical profession extended its public health work far beyond its attack on the great white plague. Many medical societies realized that compulsory attendance laws practically required the adoption of inspection measures and called for medical inspection in public schools. Although Sweden introduced an inspection system in 1840, Paris in 1843, and numerous other European nations and cities several decades later, only eight American cities and no states had provided for inspection by 1900. Boston led with a plan inaugurated in 1894, Chicago followed in 1895, New York in 1896, and Philadelphia two years later.[15]

The movement for medical inspection, which had as its original

goal the prevention of the spread of contagious diseases, broadened
its objectives after the new century began. In 1903 the Ophthalmolog-
ical Section of the American Medical Association urged that school
authorities, state legislators, and boards of health and of education
unite to secure examination of the eyes and ears of schoolchildren.
Cornelius C. Wholey a Pittsburgh physician, suggested that efforts
should be made to detect any other mental or physical defects and to
investigate the hygienic condition of the school environment.[16] Later,
Fletcher B. Dressler, a specialist in school hygiene, told the National
Education Association at its 1912 Chicago session that inspection should
be especially concerned with detection of defects that caused permanent
injury when not promptly corrected. When the Spartanburg Medical
Society of South Carolina provided inspection of the city's schools,
its program included the detection of parasitic infections. In 1910,
New Jersey became the first state to provide for general physical examinations in schools.[17]

Just as inspection plans differed in scope and emphasis, they differed also in their administrative provisions. In several states only
cities established inspection programs. In 1911, Pennsylvania provided an inspection system administered by the board of education for
first-, second-, and third-class districts, while placing whatever inspection rural areas secured under the supervision of the state board of
health. The Massachusetts law of 1907 placed enforcement of medical
inspection upon the board of education except in cities where responsibility fell wholly upon the state health board. The laws in Vermont and
Connecticut followed the Massachusetts pattern. In Illinois and New
York general responsibility lay with the state boards of health, while
state educational boards assumed responsibility of inspection for eye,
ear, and nose defects in Texas, Minnesota, Kansas, and Montana. In some
localities medical societies alone took responsibility for this service.[18]

The medical profession has left several descriptions of its contributions to inspection programs. Although a New Orleans public health
official recalled that some physicians opposed the inspection plan the
city introduced in 1908, they generally supported such programs. Cincinnati required that applicants pass civil service examinations to
qualify for employment, and the city faced no recruitment shortage.
It denied inspectors an opportunity to engage in private practice or to
render treatment and required that school authorities entrust parents
with responsibility for securing treatment of their defective or ailing

children, which often resulted in no treatment. Medical inspectors often followed rigid if not rigorous schedules. In Manhattan, doctors arrived between 8:30 and 9:10 each morning of the school week to search for contagious diseases. A new plan of inspection that New York City adopted in 1902 required not only morning inspection but weekly examinations in which inspectors gave special attention to children in kindergartens and early grades.[19]

The inspection movement made rapid progress in the decade before World War I through the united efforts of private physicians and public health officials. Oscar Dowling, president of the Louisiana State Board of Health, exemplifies the best leadership in the crusade. Early in the second decade he issued two hundred fifty thousand monthly bulletins to schoolchildren stressing the importance of inspection and hoping through students to reach their parents. By 1914 twenty states and over four hundred cities had established programs, but the movement fell short of its goals and rural areas in particular were neglected. Furthermore, some state statutes made inspection permissible rather than compulsory, and by 1908 only New Jersey's law provided for compulsory treatment. Six years later a New Orleans health official declared with some exaggeration that the inspection movement had not passed beyond the infant stage and added that no state had an adequate inspection law.[20]

PURE MILK CRUSADE

The profession's public health struggle took on even greater significance when it added a pure milk crusade to its campaign against the spread of tuberculosis and for school inspection. Although the profession found allies in the struggle, it could take most of the credit for the modest accomplishments in advancing this reform. When Henry L. Coit, a Newark physician, brought the strength of the Essex County Medical Society behind his effort to create a Medical Milk Commission in 1892, his work led not only to the formation of a local commission but to a national organization as well. Furthermore, he introduced the term "certified milk," which served as a slogan for the movement and as a copyrighted label imposing high standards on dairies that sought its use.[21]

Cincinnati became one of the major cities to adopt inspection as the movement spread westward. In 1906 the local Academy of Medicine authorized the appointment of a milk commission, which in turn called for a conference that convened at Atlantic City 3 June 1907 to establish a national body. The 125 physicians from twenty-two cities who attended this meeting quickly organized the American Association of Medical Milk Commissioners, which drafted a set of uniform inspection standards. By 1910, fifty-eight medical societies had established milk commissions that assumed either full or partial responsibility for milk inspection, while three states, New York, Kentucky, and New Jersey, had passed measures implementing patent rights by protecting the "certified milk" label.[22]

Probably no state association surpassed the California society in its crusade for milk inspection. The society authorized the creation of a Pure Food Commission at the 1906 annual session, which immediately took up a problem that the editor of the state society's journal described as "the filthy and disgraceful condition of our milk supply."[23] By 1909 the certified milk industry had developed so rapidly that the state society formed the California Association of Medical Milk Commissions, which held regular meetings at the society's annual sessions. Composed of milk commissions of county societies, the state organization sought to publicize the merits of certified milk by public meetings and lectures and by the circulation of literature. The Los Angeles County Commission put forth even greater efforts. It got the city board of health to adopt a score card for inspection prepared by the United States Department of Agriculture and, with the health board, prevailed upon the city council to increase the number of inspectors from two to eight. The council authorized inspectors to investigate all dairies, even in other counties, from which Los Angeles received its milk supply. In August 1907 the *Journal of the California State Medical Society* reported that two physicians on the State Pure Food Commission had joined the city's health officers on two dairy inspection tours, each covering about seventy-five miles.[24] Within another decade medical commissions in many other localities carried out their inspection functions about as enthusiastically.

PURE FOOD AND DRUG LEGISLATION

Actually the milk inspection crusade stood out as only a part of the profession's struggle to protect the public from impure food products. Medical societies had supported the enactment of food and drugs laws that many states passed, but these measures were weak or ineffective or both. Guided by the leadership of the AMA, they called for the improvement of state legislation along lines established by the model bill that the AMA had endorsed and circulated in 1909. They frequently rendered immeasurable assistance to state health boards in publicizing the extent of food adulteration reported by these agencies. When J. N. Hurtz, Indiana chemist and sanitarian, exposed food adulteration there in 1904, the state society told physicians that he had found 47 percent of 191 samples adulterated. Moreover, many state journals waged unremitting warfare on the patent medicine industry. Although the *Journal of the American Medical Association* launched the profession's fight against nostrum advertising, the *California State Journal of Medicine* rivaled the national organ in its demand for government control over the production of food and drugs and surpassed it in its haste to strike nostrum advertisements from its pages.[25]

The medical profession took a belated interest in agitation for federal pure food and drugs legislation, but acted soon enough to support its passage in 1906. The AMA brought its national machinery into operation, including a network of committees in many states that exerted the profession's influence directly on members of Congress. In the closing stages of debate, physicians flooded Congress with countless letters urging passage of the measure. That 865 of the first thousand judgments under the national law pertained to food adulteration indicated the medical profession's contribution to the struggle for uncontaminated food in interstate trade. Furthermore, it implemented the government's efforts to deal with nostrums under the drug provisions of the law by its relentless crusade against medical quackery and its contribution to federal investigations.[26]

EXTENSION OF REFORMS

Medical societies exerted their influence less vigorously in several other areas of reform. Deploring the ravages of ophthalmia neonatorum, which caused blindness in more than 29 percent of the residents in twenty state institutions devoted to the care of the blind, medical societies supported legislation requiring employment of simple and effective procedures at childbirth to prevent these tragedies. Medical organizations could take much credit for the passage of such laws in twenty-five states by 1911. In attempting to prevent employment of unlicensed midwives, or of any at all, they also hoped to reduce the the incidence of puerperal infection.[27]

When New York State established the first laboratory in the world devoted to cancer research at Buffalo in 1899 it raised the hopes of a profession that often lost in its struggle with a major killer. The founding of the American Association for Cancer Research in New York City in 1907 testified to the survival of these hopes. Attacking a mysterious and elusive enemy, medical societies used the meager resources at their command. They established cancer commissions to investigate the peril and devoted an entire issue of their journals in July 1915 to discussions of the problem. Among physicians they emphasized methods of early detection and in the second decade conducted a crusade to alert the public to the symptoms and the dangers of cancer.[28]

More confidently, medical societies fought diseases that yielded to advances in vaccination, inoculation, and measures of sanitation. They joined with other health organizations to inform the public, long terrorized by what had become controllable diseases, of a new day in preventive medicine. Some physicians and societies took action to see that the benefits of preventive medicine reached lower economic classes. In Indiana in 1907 a physician and legislator, J. Frank Simison, secured passage of a bill drafted by the state health department providing free antitoxin for impoverished families. Five years later the president of the Alabama society announced approvingly that the state recently had made free diphtheria antitoxin available to the poor. The law, however, required a doctor's written confirmation of medical indigency.[29] The New York state society's Committee on Public Health urged that the government's laboratory make all of the vaccine used in the state and supply all who needed it free of charge or at cost, which sometimes was no more than one-tenth the market price. Few societies carried their agitation this far, but most supported local efforts to protect public health by securing pure water supplies and adequate sewage and waste disposal systems. Several state societies worked to secure the establishment of state pathological laboratories that were important to the public and to many physicians. The Georgia medical association proposed that the state appropriate one-half of the funds from the dog tax for the support of such agencies.[30]

MATTERS OF EUGENICS

The medical societies that worked the hardest to advance measures of public health sometimes cast greatest doubt on the achievements possible through this approach. In an era when hordes of immigrants provoked nativistic prophecies of "race suicide" some medical societies sounded an alarm over propagation by the unfit. Indeed, the "Indiana Movement" that started in the first decade drew much of its support from physicians.

In 1905 the legislature of Indiana passed a law prohibiting persons with venereal diseases, epileptics, imbeciles, and those of unsound mind under guardianships from marrying. Supplementing this legislation, a physician and legislator, Horace G. Read, secured enactment of a sterilization law two years later, which Harry C. Sharp, a physician of the Indiana reformatory at Jeffersonville, had proposed. This measure allowed sterilization of confirmed criminals, rapists, imbeciles, and idiots when a medical advisory board created by the law found the condition of such inmates irremediable and recommended the procedure. During the first year Sharp sterilized 412 inmates. The Committee on State Medicine of the Indiana society considered the act "in accord with our best knowledge, and with the scientific handling of such problems." The *Southern Medical Journal* declared bluntly that the legal penalty inflicted by the sterilization of rapists would have a more "salutary" effect, especially in the South, "than many lynchings and even burnings at the stake." By 1910 at least six states had followed the Indiana plan in regulating marriage, and several others, including California, Connecticut, Oregon, and Utah, had adopted comparable sterilization laws. The legislative Committee of the Texas association endorsed the purpose of a law preventing the marriage of persons with any one of various afflictions, but believed that public opinion would not support such legislation.[31]

AGITATION FOR VITAL STATISTICS LAWS

Much to the dismay of the medical profession, the public not only was apathetic toward matters of health, but was unconcerned about the collection of statistical data that would reveal its own plight. The states' methods of collecting vital statistics were little better than procedures used by Hawaii and Puerto Rico when the United States added these islands to its empire at the end of the century. States that took regular counts of oysters, game, and terrapins and that weighted their files with records of pedigreed horses, cats, dogs, and cows often kept no record of human offspring. In 1901 only ten states (all in the North and Northeast) and the District of Columbia had mortality statistics that met the modest standards of the federal census bureau. In the South, Louisiana, for example, kept no birth and mortality statistics whatever before 1900, except in New Orleans and Shreveport, and to a lesser extent in Baton Rouge. Alabama, where responsibility for collection fell on county medical societies, had a better but far from perfect system.[32]

The American Public Health Association led the movement for adequate vital statistics laws, but many medical societies provided invaluable support. Major medical journals kept the issue before state societies whose spokesmen frequently pressed their case on state legislatures. The American Medical Association assisted by preparing a model bill for state adoption and worked vigorously with constituent societies to secure its passage. Late in the first decade, Joseph N. McCormack joined Cressy L. Wilbur, chief statistician of the Bureau of the Census, and the two pressed the matter in addresses before the legislatures of Missouri and Kansas.[33]

The movement had made considerable progress by 1910. Five additional states met the census requirement for mortality records in 1906, and four more had legislation in force by 1911. Although these gains were impressive, George W. Webster, president of the Illinois State Board of Health, charged in that year that not a single state provided for complete registration of births and that none collected adequate mortality statistics. Even though administrative inadequacies retarded progress in some states, by 1913 twenty-two had fallen within the national registration area. Nor did the war years and early aftermath obstruct many others in the adoption of the AMA's model bill or some close approximation. Two years after the war ended the AMA reported that only five states had failed to adopt such legislation.[34]

NATIONAL HEALTH DEPARTMENT ISSUE

Recognizing that the nation's growth and its scientific progress had blurred state boundaries, medical societies called for a national health department equipped to deal with problems beyond the reach of state health agencies. Led by the American Medical Association, they gave greater attention to this matter than to any other national issue in the last half of the Progressive Era. As early as 1906 the AMA had insisted upon the creation of a federal department with cabinet status, though later it sometimes wavered and was ready to settle for less. At the annual session of 1908 it chose McCormack to present the case for a health department to members of the Sixtieth Congress. Immediately he appealed to local societies for support, proposing that they appoint two committees composed of members of the two major political parties who would inquire into the views of their congressional candidates on the health department issue. McCormack made little headway either among societies or at the nation's capital and soon left Washington in disgust.[35]

When Senator Robert L. Owen of Oklahoma introduced a national health department bill in 1910, the profession's hopes for the establishment of a department quickly revived. After the first measure died in the Senate Committee on Public Health and Quarantine, Owen introduced another bill on 6 April 1911. Apparently to hasten the passage of the second bill, he omitted reference to cabinet status for the health department. Willing to compromise, the AMA and its constituent societies gave the measure enthusiastic support. The AMA's Council on Health and Public Instruction urged some two thousand members of the association's National Auxiliary Legislative Committee to support the bill and to write their congressmen to secure its passage. Many state and regional medical associations brought their journals into the fight, urging physicians to press the issue upon their congressmen and senators.[36]

But as the AMA exerted mounting pressure, implacable opposition rose from several sources. Albert F. Stephens, a prominent eclectic physician, charged that the AMA sought to establish a medical monopoly and to exclude from federal service any physician who did not have the "brand of allopathy burned into his hide."[37] William N. Mundy, editor of the principal eclectic journal, contended that the bill made way for a paternalistic government controlled by a political machine. The National Institute of Homeopathy tried to forestall the AMA by appointing its own committee to draft a bill and later by proposing that the task be assigned to a conference of commissioners already appointed by the governors of forty states to consider uniform state legislation. The Christian Science movement joined these medical groups in opposition to the bill, while patent medicine manufacturers vented their wrath through their own front organization, the National League for Medical Freedom.[38]

As it fought off assaults of insurgency within Republican ranks, the Taft administration barely placated some segments of the public health movement by supporting legislation creating a Children's Bureau early in 1912. Since most medical leaders had been largely indifferent to this issue they were not appeased and pressed their claims for a health department on the major parties as they prepared

for the presidential campaign a few months later. When the Democratic Convention adopted a platform that included a strong plank for
a national health department, the *Journal of the American Medical
Association* told physicians that it had virtually endorsed the second
Owen bill. Yet Democratic victory in November left physicians little
room for hope. Owen's second bill died in committee, and the new
administration failed to support the third bill, which he introduced on
7 April 1913. Finding other matters more pressing, President Woodrow
Wilson did not include a national health department on his agenda
of reform.[39]

III MATTERS OF ECONOMICS

CHAPTER SEVEN

DOCTORS' DILEMMA: Combining Professional Welfare and Public Interest

American physicians got little sympathy from the public when they aired their economic grievances early in the twentieth century. Since laymen seldom viewed medical practice as an avenue to wealth and probably preferred that physicians struggle on the fringes of poverty, they usually either ignored their plight or seemed annoyed by the volume of their complaints. When the profession's recruitment crusade stressed the improvement of its economic status, critics noted that the profession's policies closely resembled those of monopolies and trusts. Striking comparisons also could have been drawn from the Middle Ages when trade and merchant guilds restricted entry into business, controlled the conditions of admission, exercised discipline over members, and set minimum wages for their labor and minimum prices for their products. But in an era when the public read repeated exposures of monopolistic designs, the profession's critics did not need to venture far into the past to find precedents for its policies.[1]

ECONOMIC RATIONALE

Leaders of the medical profession paid little attention to their critics and found ways to reconcile the professional ideal of service with the concept of group interest. Convinced that the financial stress felt by many physicians diminished their competence in practice, Joseph N. McCormack told the Tennessee State Medical Association in 1904 that "the time has come in the history of medicine when the doctor who is a failure financially, is necessarily a failure as a medical man."[2] He did not intend to imply that professional success could be measured in financial terms, but that the conditions of practice in the twentieth century had begun to place unusual economic burdens on the profession. Higher costs of medical training, growing demands of continuous education, more costly outlays for facilities, and general inflationary pressures made the profession's concern for its economic welfare a question of survival. And while physicians saw the growing demands of practice place greater strains on their budgets, they also watched advances in preventive medicine reduce the incidences of illness as an oversupply of medical schools turned out graduates to compete for the cases that remained.[3]

TRACKS OF THE TRUST

In an effort to reduce competition and to elevate and stabilize income, the American Medical Association introduced or revived in the professional world policies that monopolistic enterprise had employed successfully in the world of business. Hardly had the United States Steel Corporation succeeded in its consolidation efforts that raised prices of basic steel products in 1901 from 200 or 300 percent above the more competitive level of 1898 when the medical profession began its income uplift and price maintenance program. Societies that never had adopted fee schedules and others that had left their schedules unchanged for decades quickly brought their professional fees in line with the inflationary trends of the Progressive Era.[4]

As the medical profession began to price its services in much the same way industrial combines set their prices, it had to consider the application of legislation designed to control business enterprise that it once had ignored. Nor could it overlook the possibility that an aroused public would strengthen laws adequately to cover a professional monopoly. When Kansas led the way in 1889 with the first general legislation regulating trusts, it specifically prohibited price setting and fee schedules by lawyers and doctors.[5] Seven other states hastily secured trust legislation before Congress passed the Sherman Antitrust Act of 1890, but without specific reference to professional practices. Whether by statute or by constitutional amendment, twenty-nine states took action to place some kind of control over monopolistic enterprise before the century ended.[6]

In moving toward price fixing and price maintenance, the profession, more than industrial combinations, risked still another chance of arousing public protest. Although the American medical profession used fee schedules in the Colonial Era, it never convinced the public that price fixing was a legitimate professional function. Furthermore, tradition, readily acknowledged in colonial times, allowed public regulation, especially in areas of inelastic demand. A law of the Plymouth Colony in 1638 forbade "engrossing," "regrading," or "oppressing" buyers "when their necessyties do constrain them to buy at any price," and another, enacted by the Virginia House of Burgesses the next year, allowed an appeal to the county court for persons charging physicians with extortion in pricing drugs and medical services. Still another Virginia law, in 1662, placed the financial aspects of professional practice under public supervision, and the enactment of a maximum fee schedule for doctors about seventy-five years later showed that the colony had not surrendered public control over the economic policies of physicians.[7]

Whether the public would revive the colonial practice of imposing restraints on a profession seeking economic advancement by collective effort remained in doubt early in the new century. Physicians got none of the specific exemptions that a few state laws accorded to industrial workers, whose labor was not a "commodity" within the meaning of these measures. The greatest comfort they received came from sluggish enforcement of the legislation in some states and from the total absence of such statutes in others.[8]

The real or potential threat of antitrust legislation stood as only one impediment to the efforts of physicians to achieve price stability. In a cautious moment of restraint the profession itself raised another. During the great reorganizational effort beginning in 1901, some state associations adopted constitutions and bylaws that allowed neither these associations nor affiliated societies to issue fee schedules. The constitution of the Alabama association prohibited local societies from discussing the topic in their meetings. At first the reorganizational movement enrolled fewer than one-half of the physicians in some areas, and county societies declined to establish fee schedules to which only a portion of the profession would adhere.[9]

COURT ENCOUNTERS

Neither the threat of antitrust prosecution nor the constitutional provisions against price fixing prevented the profession from framing fee schedules in most states. At best it only slowed the process. In 1907 the Texas association boldly published the fee schedules of eighty-nine county societies after the attorney general of the state ruled that their price-fixing activity was not prohibited by the state antitrust law, which exempted organizations formed for the purpose of protecting labor, "manual or mental or both." Physicians in Iowa had reason to rejoice when in 1907 a trial court in Bremer County declared that their price-fixing agreement did not conflict with the anti-trust law (*W. A. Rohlf* v. *Henry Kasemeier and the State of Iowa*) in a decision that the state supreme court soon upheld. This appeal court affirmed that the state did not prohibit price-fixing agreements involving labor, skilled or unskilled, which was not a "commodity" within the meaning of the law.[10]

The Kansas profession found that it could move with no such boldness. In May 1906 the Kansas City *Times* reported that the state attorney general, C. C. Coleman, had instructed A. J. Freeborn, attorney of Washington County, to begin prosecution of twenty-five doctors who had organized a society and agreed upon a fee schedule. Coleman told Freeborn that such an agreement violated the law even if the society attached no penalties for breaking the fee scale and that he should prosecute officers of the "trust" and each doctor who entered into the agreement. John C. Rudolph, a physician of Hanover, Kansas, probably expressed the professional sentiment of the state when he bitterly protested, "Shall the physicians of Kansas be the only wage earners, who are excluded by law and shall a union of physicians be declared by any light headed law-twister a trust! That may happen in Russia—but it will not happen in the 'land of the free and the home of the brave.' "[11] Washington County physicians did not walk into danger without receiving a word of warning. In 1904 the editor of their state society's journal cited the Kansas law and, while disclaiming any intention of employing the techniques of "present-day unionism," he suggested that physicians "should so meet together and compare notes that our fees as well as our dealings with the public may be consistent and proportionate to the demands made upon us."[12]

In some cases the Kansas statute served to restrain physicians from drawing up fee schedules, and in others it probably caused them only to proceed quietly with the effort. No statutes specifically outlawing such schedules existed, however, in other states. In these the most effective deterrents came from a fear that the public, once aroused, might secure legislation prohibiting price-fixing practices, or that it would turn to irregular physicians for medical care. Regular physicians sought to prevent retaliatory legislation by secretly adopting or raising fee schedules, and they tried to prevent widespread recourse to irregular practitioners by appealing to them, sometimes successfully, to adhere to the standard.[13]

SPORADIC PROTESTS

The Piatt County Medical Society in Illinois faced troubles typical of medical groups that ignored elementary rules of secrecy in drawing up their schedules. Public violence almost occurred when the society gave newspaper publicity to its fee revisions in 1906. At Cerro Gordo enraged citizens held a mass meeting, passed resolutions condemning price fixing, and threatened to boycott local physicians and import others. But county physicians held out against the public only in this normally peaceful town. Elsewhere in the county, N. L. Barker, secretary of the society, reported, "This little test has served to show that some of the members of the profession in this county have very, very weak quadriceps extensors and that the contractile power of the extensor muscles of the lower extremities has been absorbed by the flexor muscle of the same." Thus describing the profession's retreat before the public's attack he admonished, "never give publicity to the fee-bills, for the people will not appreciate what was intended for kindness and justice. Make your fees and let them go quietly into effect. Then the opposition will not be so united."[14] Physicians of Williamsport, Pennsylvania, soon could attest to the wisdom of his warning when the public responded to an announcement of a fee increase with a successful boycott and by recourse to the services of doctors outside the city.[15]

Physicians had much to fear from probing newspaper editors and special interest groups. When doctors of Greene County, Illinois, raised their fees in the middle of the decade, an editor of an adjoining county attempted to arouse the public by branding their organization a medical trust. When physicians in Carbondale, Pennsylvania, raised their fees for office consultation from twenty-five to fifty cents, labor unions responded by proposing the importation of other doctors, only to be charged by a local physician with threatening to use "scab" labor. So intense became the conflict that the society appealed unsuccessfully to Joseph N. McCormack to intervene.[16]

Although the introduction of price fixing brought turbulence in some areas, the profession succeeded in preventing popular outbursts far more often than it failed. Medical journals of the era reported many cases of fee-schedule adoptions, but seldom indicated that they brought public protest. That a large portion of medical societies over the nation adopted or updated fee schedules in the Progressive Era seems fairly certain although much of the evidence never reached the medical press. That a considerable number of physicians sought society membership in order to use the organization for economic advancement also seems clear. McCormack, in his recruitment crusade, often failed to reach doctors on an idealistic level and he deplored their widespread indifference to the profession's noblest goals.[17]

FEE SCHEDULE GUIDE

McCormack always insisted that economic considerations should play a subordinate role in his recruitment drive. Not until 1906 did he draft a fee schedule for consideration by the profession at large, suggesting means for its implementation as well (see Appendix V). He excluded surgery from his schedule; and his fees were to serve largely as a guideline. Attempting to conform to constitutional requirements that often prohibited medical organizations from adopting price-fixing policies, he advised that the practice should be supported by *individual doctors* rather than by the society as a whole. Deploring the secrecy of societies in adopting fee schedules, he insisted that these regulations should not become effective until after public consultation, and he called for no penalties for violations other than those professional disapproval might impose.[18]

BLACKLISTING ISSUE

Medical societies not only brought their fee schedules in line with the inflationary forces of the Progressive Era, but also sought protection from patients who did not pay their bills. McCormack advised the employment of bill collectors in some instances to relieve the profession of this task. But he deplored the use of a "blacklist" against nonpaying patients, although such lists appear to have been used more than occasionally.[19] The Carlisle County (Kentucky) Medical Society serves as no isolated example of a society that employed a blacklist to deal with payment delinquency. Under penalty of expulsion from the society, members pledged to enforce the schedule and to collect from delinquent patients. The society circulated a delinquent list among its members forbidding any physician to administer medical care (except in emergencies, and then for cash payment only) until all previous accounts had been paid. In all cases, except emergencies, each physician agreed to inform any person seeking his services of any prior record of payment delinquency. Only after the prospective patient paid or arranged for payment of overdue bills with any physician in the society would he be provided with medical care. The physician receiving payment, or accepting a plan for discharging the debt, issued a certificate on a form that the society prescribed, which served as a notice to other physicians that the debt had been paid or that provision for payment had been made. If the patient failed to comply with the terms of payment as specified, the society again would place his name on the delinquent list and require that every physician "refuse absolutely" to render further service until he could provide a new certificate[20] (see Appendix VI).

PROBLEM OF FREE DISPENSARIES

Unfortunately, debt delinquency or default did not exhaust the threats raised by a portion of the public to the profession's search for economic security. To the enormous losses physicians sustained through payment evasions they added other losses attributable to the spread of free dispensaries and discount clinics. As some localities moved feebly to meet the medical needs of the disheartened and diseased segment of the population, physicians charged that they opened the doors to groups that needed no such assistance. Mounting evidence supported their claim that not least among the threats to the prosperity of private practice was the abuse of free dispensaries.

Out of the sprawling urban slums poured hordes of impoverished sufferers seeking treatment in scattered dispensaries. As the new century began, 51 percent of New York City's population bore the classification of medical paupers, and in 1905, 994,315 patients applied for free medical aid at dispensaries in the metropolitan area. Six years later Manhattan alone had 665,000 new dispensary patients, while onefourth of Chicago's population received free medical care. New Orleans was another of many cities bearing the growing burdens of medical indigency, as a resident physician complained that it had become "the dumping ground for the maimed and injured of other States!"[21]

Convinced that dispensaries often administered aid to the affluent and the poor alike, doctors in many states sought to block encroachments on their domain. They publicized accounts of wealthy citizens crowding the indigent away from dispensary doors, "clothed in fine raiment, decked with jewelry." According to this account the "Diamond Dispensary" (apparently in New York City) got its name from its gratuitous service to the rich.[22] The *Illinois Medical Journal* charged that while 25 percent of the population of Chicago received

free medical care, only one-half of 1 per cent got other forms of charity. Nor did medical journals spare university hospitals from attack.
The *Journal of the Michigan State Medical Society* contended that the
minimal weekly charges at the University of Michigan hospital lay
beyond the reach of the poor but well within the range of undeserving classes who exploited the system. "Underbidding for business," the
editorial said, "ranks low among the best merchants, because it por-
tends future disaster; for the same reason, underbidding by hospitals
or individuals has created an atmosphere antagonistic to their highest
usefulness."[23]

Physicians condemning the dispensary abuse usually could only
guess at its scope and the extent of its danger. The scant resources
of their societies allowed for no costly and extensive surveys. Not until
1912 did the findings of a major canvass reach the medical press, and
this survey offered little confirmation of the profession's fears. In 1911
a subcommittee of the Committee on Dispensary Abuse of the Medical
Society of the County of New York chose Anne Moore, an expert social
worker with a doctoral degree, to conduct a survey based on the
665,000 new cases in which Manhattan dispensaries administered
treatment in that year. She selected 1,000 cases at random for close
investigation. Unable to locate 255 patients in the sample, she drew
her conclusions from her study of the economic conditions of 745.
Of this number, she found 672, or 90 percent, who seemed deserving
of free treatment. Furthermore, she concluded, "The average poor
family can not afford sickness and what it entails. It can barely afford
the necessities that sustain life when wage earners are working to
capacity."[24]

Medical societies frequently complained of the dispensary abuse
and less often took action against it. The Boston Medical Society protested bitterly to the superintendents and trustees of the city's hospitals in 1910 over the alleged practice of allowing "indiscriminating
medical charity." A year later the Council of the Chicago Medical
Society announced adoption of a plan to combine all free dispensaries of the city with United Charities in an effort to eliminate what it
thought was a growing evil. The plan called for the investigation of
the economic condition of every person seeking free treatment.[25]

Disturbed by an abuse it could not stop, the medical profession
sought the power of the state to implement action. The New York
statute of 1899 contained most of the features the profession hoped

to incorporate in such legislation. This statute placed the control of dispensaries under the State Board of Charities and required the posting of the law in a dispensary and the appointment of a registrar to supervise its work, control the admission of all applicants, and preserve their records. Fines of as much as $250 could be imposed on persons securing treatment under false representation, and a jail penalty might be attached until the fine was paid. When the Pennsylvania Medical Society sought enactment of a similar law two years later, the *Journal of the American Medical Association* approved the action but contended that societies in states enacting such legislation should prepare to check dispensary records to ensure enforcement.[26] Despite the restrictions imposed by some dispensaries and the persistence of professional agitation, medical societies seldom believed that they had been effective in curbing the dispensary abuses of the early twentieth century.

BATTLE WITH DRUGGISTS

As physicians fought free dispensaries that attracted prospective patients, they also guarded the medical domain against throngs of invading druggists. They long had condemned druggists who used substitutes in filling prescriptions, but other practices of pharmacists were more important in widening the gap of estrangement between the two professions in the Progressive Era. They attacked pharmacists for counterprescribing, for refilling prescriptions without authorization, and for recommending patent medicines, while pharmacists, in turn, attacked the medical profession for drug dispensing.[27]

Physicians rightly protested the widespread practice of counterprescribing, but knew that within their own ranks the neglect of therapeutic instruction had encouraged the trend. When both medical schools and the profession lost most of their interest in materia medica in this age of therapeutic nihilism, a drug-seeking population often turned to pharmacists through physicians' default. Nevertheless, medical leaders deplored the trend and recognized the dangers. Speaking at the annual session of the American Pharmaceutical Association in September 1907, McCormack charged that "druggists and their boy clerks" administered primary treatment for 50 to 75 percent of the gonorrhea cases in most sections of the nation and that the same percentage of operative surgery performed on women annually could be traced to the futile attempts of drugstores to treat this disease.[28]

Other prominent physicians joined McCormack in his attack on the counterprescription abuse. Julius H. Comroe of York, Pennsylvania, charged that it had become "probably the greatest and most criminal" of all the outrages inflicted on the public by the profession of pharmacy and called it a "criminal abuse of the practice of medicine." Lloyd A. Clary, a Kansas physician, declared that many doctors had resorted to dispensing in retaliation against druggists who usurped their function by counterprescribing. The *Journal of the Missouri State Medical Association* cited an opinion of the state assistant health commissioner that such procedure violated the state's medical practice act.[29] Indeed, as medical societies secured provisions in medical practice laws that broadened the definition of practice to include, at least implicitly, counterprescribing, they probably exercised their greatest influence against the abuse.

The unauthorized refilling of prescriptions was another widespread pharmaceutical abuse against which physicians made frequent protest. Few doctors complained when, with no instructions to the contrary, pharmacists refilled prescriptions once or twice. But they criticized the persistent issuance of drugs extending even over a period of years under the same prescription. A Pennsylvania physician discovered that one of his prescriptions had circulated "with little rest" for two decades. Another observed that patients praising remedies prescribed by their doctors occasionally loaned their bottles to ailing neighbors who secured refills. And, too, the profession charged that pharmacists often paid no attention to the instructions forbidding a refill when they appeared clearly on the prescription.[30]

Physicians offered proposals to eliminate the prescription-refilling abuse but to no avail. Charles E. Seiver, a Kansas physician, told the state medical association that legislatures should enact laws that would protect the public against this evil. He suggested that such laws should require pharmacists, upon filling prescriptions, to mark them canceled and, after holding a prescription for forty days, to return it to the issuing physician. Yet legislation restricting pharmacists was not passed. Instead powerful pharmaceutical interests secured legislation, at least in North Dakota, that prevented doctors from dispensing at all except in cases of emergency.[31]

While counterprescribing and the unauthorized refilling of prescriptions strained relations between the medical and pharmaceutical professions in the Progressive Era, the problem of patent medicines became the most divisive issue. As the profession sought to drive proprietary advertising from its journals and to strike nostrums from the prescription lists of physicians, it also attacked the drugstores as a major conduit of quackery. In fact, counterprescribing thrived on the nostrum racket, and a substantial part of the income of pharmacists came from this source.

McCormack insisted that the success of the nostrum industry depended totally on the unholy alliance it had established with the news media and the drug trade. He charged that the alliance had become a powerful political force. After carrying his public health crusade to many state capitals, often addressing legislative bodies, he told the American Pharmaceutical Association that he found powerful "drug men," supported by the proprietary interests and directed by skilled lobbyists of the National Association of Retail Druggists, fighting passage of food and drugs legislation at every capital he visited. Legislators, he charged, were "literally inundated by letters and telegrams from their drug and newspaper constituents in the interests of these now fully exposed and recognized frauds." Professing his genuine appreciation of pharmacists and his commitment to the "prescription method of dispensing," he confessed that "the discovery of the almost universal ascendancy of the quack interests over the trade was a painful one."[32] Declaring that the two professions apparently had reached "the parting of the ways," he warned that physicians must take over their own dispensing if such differences between the medical and pharmaceutical professions remained.[33]

Unfortunately, McCormack could not speak for a united profession on the patent medicine issue. As he well knew, the nostrum industry had sharply divided the ranks of medicine and had lured a large part of the profession because it thrived on the nostrum prescriptions issued by physicians. Edward Bok probably surprised the public far more than the medical profession when he examined five thousand prescriptions from the files of Philadelphia drugstores in 1905 and announced that 41 percent called for compounds of unknown content.[34] Two years later, when physicians of Bowling Green, Kentucky, pledged to prescribe only by the *United States Pharmacopoeia* and the *National Formulary,* all the pharmacists in town wired frantically for drugs to fill their orders. "Certainly," declared Arthur T. McCormack, a physician and son of the distinguished organizer, "no further comment is needed to show the condition to which the medical and pharmaceutical professions have been reduced by the growth of the nostrum evil."[35] Even in the home town of the McCormacks many physicians only recently had severed connections with the nostrum trade.

The skirmish with pharmacists over the nostrum issue rates only as a minor phase of a major fight. On the national front the profession, detecting the magnitude of the menace, united its ranks for its fourth and hardest battle. Seldom did the struggle against the economic encroachments of druggists and dispensaries, or with the public over such matters as debt default, develop the enmity aroused by its attack on the nostrum trade.

ANTINOSTRUM STRUGGLE

Upon the American Medical Association fell the heaviest burden of the conflict, but a number of state societies gave substantial aid. The national association waged an attack upon the patent medicine empire on various fronts throughout the Progressive Era. It attempted, with a growing measure of success, to drive nostrum advertisements from the pages of medical publications. Through the work of the newly created Council on Pharmacy and Chemistry, which investigated all compounds submitted by companies designed for physicians' practice, it attempted to combat the evils of nostrum prescription. In its struggle for national food and drugs legislation and for the enactment of similar laws in all of the states it tried with some success to extend effective government regulation over the proprietary industry. And finally, after the enactment of federal legislation, the American Medical Association carried on a crusade throughout the nation to alert the public to the dangers of nostrum use.

The victories won by the medical profession over the patent medicine interests mark some of the profession's most significant achievements in the Progressive Era. For the first time the forces of quackery fell back in disarray. The alliance between the nostrum manufacturers, druggists, and the press was greatly weakened and the public became better informed on rational approaches to problems of health. In addition, the AMA had raised the image of a profession widely held in disesteem and had struck at a serious economic threat. Out of more than a decade of warfare came experience useful to the profession as it confronted the nostrum menace in newer forms in later decades.[36]

SURVIVAL OF MIDWIFERY

A fifth issue disturbing the profession in the Progressive Era gave rise to much greater protests in some areas than in others. As obstetrics made faltering moves toward specialty status, agitation rose over the persistence of midwifery, which the profession increasingly felt did not belong in the twentieth century. Not only did physicians attribute high infant mortality rates to midwifery, but they also held the ignorance of midwives chiefly responsible for infant blindness (ophthalmia neonatorum) that an application of a silver nitrate solution to the eyes of an infant at birth easily could prevent. Furthermore, they recognized the economic losses the profession suffered because midwives attended about one-half of all births in the United States in 1910 and annually diverted from the profession an income that one prominent physician estimated at $5 million three years later.[37]

Physicians followed no uniform policy in dealing with midwifery, but their goal was the passage of legislation outlawing the practice. In 1900 the Committee on Legislation of the Medical Society of the State of New York fought a bill that called for the creation of a board of examiners in midwifery for New York City, contending that the function of midwives fell within the practice of medicine and should be performed only by regular physicians. Yet a year later the New Orleans Parish Medical Society adopted a resolution simply urging the State Board of Medical Examiners to require that midwives receive proper instruction about the nature and treatment of the disease.[38] Early in the new century realistic physicians warned that no amount of opposition would defeat so entrenched a system. Maurice J. Lewi, secretary of the New York State Board of Medical Examiners, showed that in 1901 midwives reported 38,482 of the 80,735 births in New York City and that the profession could expect no more than legislation raising their licensing standards. "We are confronted," he said, "with a condition not a theory."[39]

The threat of midwifery to the profession began to decline late in the Progressive Era, but for reasons partially beyond the control of physicians and through no clear demonstration of their obstetrical superiority. In fact, the record of midwives in New York City in preventing stillbirths and puerperal sepsis surpassed that of physicians early in the second decade. In Washington, D.C., midwife deliveries declined from 50 to 15 percent in the decade after 1903, but infant mortality for the first day, first week, and first month actually increased. The teaching of obstetrics in some medical schools improved, but instruction in most institutions remained inadequate. Unexpected developments assisted physicians in resisting encroachments on their obstetrical domain. Just as immigration to the United States had flooded many areas with midwives, its curtailment during World War I reduced their inflow. Furthermore, women who pressed persistently for voting rights raised social demands as well. They appeared less willing to accept ordinary midwife care and placed pressure on major parties for federal legislation dealing with maternal and child welfare problems soon after the Progressive Era closed.[40]

CHAPTER EIGHT

CONTRACT PRACTICE

American medical practice in the early twentieth century felt the impact of economic and social forces that already had changed much of the national scene. Urbanization had gone far toward destroying the dominance of agricultural life, industrialization clouded the landscape of most of the nation's cities, and the 15.5 million immigrants who reached American shores from the beginning of the century to World War I tested the expansive capacities of the economic system. These forces made new demands upon physicians and brought into question the adequacy of the traditional medical structure and its rigid pattern of payment for medical care.

ORIGIN OF CONTRACT PRACTICE

Contract practice stood out in the Progressive Era as the most dangerous threat to whatever degree of unity the regular medical profession had achieved. This type of practice took many forms, but essentially it repudiated the traditional fee-for-service arrangement, substituting instead a system that survived on per capita assessments. In other cases it called for the employment of salaried physicians who contracted to perform an indefinite volume of work for a definite amount of pay. American experience with the system reached back to its employment in the plantation economy of the Colonial Era. It survived in relative obscurity before the Civil War, shifted largely to an urban base late in the nineteenth century, and expanded greatly before 1900.[1]

Contract practice in the railroad, mining, and logging industries established firm roots in American society late in the nineteenth century. Large industrial corporations in many cities had launched experiments with similar schemes that began to show all the signs of permanence early in the Progressive Era. Contractual plans included those established by sick and indemnity companies, which spread widely over the states, and the plans of a variety of fraternal and benevolent orders in the cities. They included the plans employed by individual hospitals and others advanced by organizations known as hospital associations. Furthermore, federal agencies sometimes adopted contract plans providing medical service for their employees, and numerous counties and cities took recourse to the contract system for giving their indigent medical care.[2]

ERA OF EXPANSION

Contract schemes were used widely in the railroad network, in the ore extractive industries of Pennsylvania, Minnesota, Michigan, Tennessee, and Alabama, and among logging companies of the Northwest. Falling largely into one class, they differed chiefly in their methods of financing. They grew out of the hazardous working conditions in these industries and the legal risks imposed by such hazards. Furthermore, the sprawling character of the railroad industry and the isolation of many mining and logging companies often required the maintenance of hospitals and demanded reliable medical service that private practice could not always provide. Only plans offering the service of salaried physicians, and in the case of railroads, supplementary agreements providing for the services of physicians along their lines, met the requirements of these industries.[3]

Neither industrial corporations nor insurance companies lost much time in exploring the advantages of contract practice. Michigan stands as an example of a leading industrial state where corporations made extensive use of this form of practice early in the new century. In 1907 the profession's survey revealed that a Benton Arbor firm operated a plan for 300 employees and that a glass plant at Saginaw brought 75 workers under similar coverage. The Michigan Alkali Company adopted a plan for 1,350 employees and the American Shipbuilding Company for 750. At Menominee the Electrical and Mechanical Company brought the coverage of contract practice to 300 more. Insurance companies with their own forms of contract practice appealed especially to firms with high industrial risks that sought to avoid the annoyance of company-administered plans. The Standard Life and Accident Insurance Company and Aetna were the major insurance organizations operating in Detroit and other major Michigan

cities.[4] Throughout the industrial North, and at scattered points elsewhere, companies offering industrial plans with contract practice
features made substantial gains.

As insurance companies moved onto the industrial front with their
contractual schemes, benevolent and fraternal orders also established
contract plans, largely among urban working classes. In large American cities many of these orders took firm root in the Progressive Era,
spreading from metropolitan areas to smaller cities and from coast
to coast. They thrived particularly in impoverished Hungarian, Polish,
Italian, and Greek sections among families who preferred the meager
medical advantages of these plans to the stigma of charity medicine.
Between 1,500 and 2,000 lodges functioned on New York's Lower
East Side, and 500 physicians had contracts with Jewish chapters.
In Buffalo the Fraternal Order of the Eagles, the Loyal Order of
Moose, and the Fraternal Order of Orioles took prominent places
among organizations covering 150,000 of its population with some form
of contract practice. In Pennsylvania the Foresters of America had 169
courts and a reported membership in Philadelphia of 30,843, but even
the growth of this organization probably was surpassed by the Fraternal Order of the Eagles in most sections of the state. The Order of
the Mystic Chain, the Independent Order of Red Men, the Brotherhood of St. John, and the Heptasophs also found Pennsylvania a favorable environment for contract practice.[5]

Fraternal orders made rapid headway in some of the East North
Central States and in parts of the upper South during the first decade.
By 1908 the Foresters claimed over 1,400 members in Pontiac, Michigan, the Eagles over 200, and the Owls, 50. The Foresters had 600
members in Bay City, 500 in Traverse City, and 400 in Lansing. By
1908 about 8,000 persons in Jackson had contract medical coverage.
Fraternal orders and some 300 independent foreign societies controlled a substantial part of the contract practice in Chicago, and
reports cited the appearance of new lodges in cities along the Ohio
River in Kentucky.[6]

Along the West Coast fraternal orders registered similar gains. By
1906 the Eagles had enrolled 3,166 members in Seattle, the Foresters,
900, the Buffaloes, 550, and the Order of Red Men, 200. Some 15,000
of its population (including dependents of enrollees) had contract
coverage from fraternal orders. These orders established groups in
California with similar ease.[7] By 1906 fraternal societies had spread

contract medical schemes throughout Los Angeles, and a little later some 10,000 of the population of San Jose had contract medical coverage. Well aware of the work of these aggressive orders, the *California State Journal of Medicine* reported that year that Foresters and Eagles had extended their organizations throughout the states.[8]

As the advance of contract schemes brought sweeping changes in medical practice, some hospitals gave way before the momentum of the movement. By 1910 over 25 percent of the hospitals of Chicago subscribed to some form of contract practice. Accepting not only individuals as beneficiaries of their services, they extended contracts to railroads, industrial corporations, and lodges as well. Ingenious promoters also organized hospital associations that sold contracts for medical care. The National Hospital Association of Portland, Oregon, and the American Hospital Association stood out within this group offering hospital and medical coverage for entire families.[9]

Government involvement in widening areas of medical care added greatly to the range of contract practice in the Progressive Era. Salaried physicians served the armed forces, staffed many posts in the United States Public Health and Marine Hospital Service, and provided medical aid to wards of the nation at government outposts. Federal hospitals for disabled veterans offered a form of contract medical care, and federal agencies at the national capital sometimes established fully equipped hospital facilities for employees. State maintenance of institutions providing medical care for disabled classes and cities bringing contract medical coverage to firemen and policemen advanced the system. Moreover, county governments, in providing a semblance of medical care for the indigent by competitive bidding, added their part to the spread of contract practice.[10]

The prospect of discount prices for medical service in an era of inflation gave contract medical schemes considerable public appeal. The promise of more stable income through contract practice made the plans particularly attractive to doctors at the marginal level of survival. Yet growing numbers of physicians saw the havoc that the system wrought to their fee schedules and price maintenance programs and predicted the economic ruin of the profession.

EXPLOITING THE PROFESSION

The degraded levels of pay under most contract practice schemes fully justified the profession's fears of exploitation. In Pennsylvania the Foresters of Reading offered physicians a per capita sum of three cents a week, while Philadelphia lodges paid only two. For the usual payment of one dollar annually the Foresters of the state offered members unlimited medical care, while the Eagles, for a normal payment of only twice this figure, gave coverage to entire families in all but obstetrical and venereal cases. Under competitive bidding procedures physicians had no assurance of getting more than a part of this amount. Though in some cases they received the entire payment, at Columbia, the Eagles assessed three dollars annually for medical care but paid physicians only from fifty to seventy-five cents.[11]

Elsewhere the outlook for the profession appeared no brighter. In Michigan, the Michigan Alkali Company provided contract coverage to employees for monthly payments of fifty cents, while at Menominee, the Electrical and Mechanical Company offered medical and surgical care for only fifteen cents. Mining corporations generally provided individual medical coverage for monthly payments of from fifty cents to one dollar, while the United States Health and Accident Company gave contract coverage in several firms for annual payments ranging from $1.50 to $3.00. Aetna Life and Accident Company provided contract coverage to a number of firms for employee payments of one dollar per month, but of this sum allowed physicians only 10 percent. Three courts of Foresters in Pontiac received coverage for annual payments of from $1.00 to $1.50, which included medicine provided by physicians. In Lima, Ohio, one fraternal order promised contract coverage for monthly payments of only sixty-five cents. Careful estimates in 1907 of the cost of contract practice in Chicago, as opposed to the cost of similar service under the minimum fee bill, set the annual loss to the profession at a minimum of $750,000.[12]

On the West Coast, the San Francisco Medical Aid Society offered family contract coverage for one dollar per month. The National Hospital Association of Portland advertised annual coverage of couples for seventeen dollars after payment of a two-dollar entrance fee. For the medical coverage provided by the Aerie of Eagles of Shasta County California, physicians received per capita payments averaging a little over sixteen cents per month. Mining and lumber companies of the county secured contract coverage for monthly payments of one dollar.[13]

Within less than a decade contract medical schemes burst from these restricted areas to embrace, indiscriminately, workers of almost any industry or trade. The medical profession could see few barriers to their expansion. As the contract practice movement gained momentum many physicians wondered if anything more than a fragment of conventional practice could be saved.

ISSUE BRINGS DIVISION

The spread of contract practice almost invariably divided the ranks of medicine. Some societies favored its employment in the railroad, ore extractive, and logging industries and by some agencies of government, but opposed its extension in other areas. This position, representing the containment principle, offered a simple solution to a troublesome issue. Arthur L. Benedict, a prominent Buffalo physician, defended this idea at a symposium of the American Academy of Medicine in 1909, when he warned against extension of contract practice but maintained that such practice among railroads, mining, and logging industries was necessary and "wholly unobjectionable."[14] By this date a majority of physicians in many medical societies held this view and opposed further extension of the system.

In a second group of societies doctors with a different opinion gained control. They neither opposed contract practice in these industries nor objected to its extension in several other areas, yet they seldom designated the legitimate limits of expansion and left the issue in much confusion. These societies received little guidance from the national association and wandered somewhat aimlessly through a bewildering variety of contract schemes. An exception was the Alabama state society, which for state organizations drew up in 1890 what appears to have been the most specific directives applied to contract practice in the Progressive Era. It recognized the legitimacy of such practice in manufacturing and mining and among tenants and hired labor on plantations. It extended contractual rights to physicians administering medical care to students attending institutions away from their homes and supported contract practice among inmates of prisons, poor farms, and charity hospitals. Furthermore, it recognized the legitimacy of contract practice for sailors and crew members in maritime trades.[15]

Some societies would have considered the directives of the Alabama association too restrictive, others too broad. Many local societies tolerated contract practice with fraternal and benevolent orders, which the Alabama association opposed. While some societies restricted the practice to railroads, mining, and logging companies, and to other industries in rare instances, the Alabama society made no such distinctions. The California State Medical Society allowed contract practice with hospital associations which the Alabama society opposed. Some societies allowed contract practice with sick and accident companies, while others forbade such extension. Few would have followed the Alabama association in extending contract practice to agricultural labor of the hired and tenant classes.[16]

PROPOSALS FOR REFORM

Although societies falling within these two groups differed widely on the legitimate limits of contract practice, they all agreed that all of its forms contained abuses. Not even contracts with railroad, mining, and logging industries escaped their criticism in the first decade. While they raised little objection to the salary level of railway surgeons, they complained that railroads issued free passes as the only reward for the services of countless physicians along their lines. Sterling D. Shimer, president of the Pennsylvania Medical Society, charged that physicians accepting passes undervalued their services even more than doctors engaged in contract practice. The *Ohio State Medical Journal* complained that railroads threw jobs at the profession in much the same way they would throw a bone to a dog.[17]

Medical societies accused railroads and mining companies of perpetuating other abuses. Under contracts that called for medical service to workmen with employment injuries, railroads often secured medical treatment for injuries not so incurred and care for families of workmen as well. Salaried officials in both the railroad and mining industries frequently got free care for themselves and their families under contracts that covered only workers, and miners received care for their dependents. Mining companies administering medical care funds created through payroll deductions often cut the earnings of physicians by retaining an excessive percentage as an administration charge.[18]

Despite frequent protests, medical societies offered only feeble resistance to these encroachments. Their complaints apparently had little effect on the policies of industries that usually could find a ready supply of physicians clamoring for their contracts. Local societies made little effort to enforce observance of their standards, and an appeal to ethics alone failed. The Alabama association gave the most

specific warnings when it declared contracts unethical that allowed
coverage of company officials and administrative charges exceeding
10 percent.[19]

Societies dominated by physicians who recognized the probable
permanence of emerging forms of contract practice sought to introduce reforms throughout the system. Their complaints and demands
were much the same whether referring to corporate plans, plans of
sick and accident insurance companies, of hospitals, or of benevolent
and fraternal orders. Watching most fearfully the spread of fraternal
and benevolent schemes and the proliferation of hospital plans, their
demands on these branches of contract practice illustrate the reforms
they sought to impose upon them all.

Medical societies raised their strongest criticism against benevolent
and fraternal orders for the meager earnings grudgingly given to physicians under service contracts. They rightfully claimed that the chief
appeal of many of these organizations was the promise of cheap medical care through the exploitation of the medical profession. In California in 1905 the Shasta County Medical Society in its struggle with
the Eagles expressed a widespread feeling when it reminded the order
that while it considered all forms of contract practice objectionable, it
had not condemned any type that "made an approach to a fair compensation." But it continued, "When our mild acceptance of a seeming
wrong encourages any lodge or society to place a valuation on our
services comparable to those of the bootblack and peanut vender and
attempts to force us into acceptance of its valuation, then indeed it is
time to feel ourselves humiliated and degraded."[20] Six years later a
committee on medical practice of the state association likewise contended that fraternal practice exploited physicians and served neither
the best interests of the profession nor of the public. But to the low-
pay problem it added the denial of the free choice of physician as
another abuse and proposed a remedy for both. It contended that "a
little more money and a retail payment of the doctor at a reasonable
rate for the work actually done, or the granting of a certain amount
of sick benefit to the individual patient, allowing him the choice of
physician, would solve the difficulty entirely."[21]

When a local court of Foresters in Providence, Rhode Island,
granted free choice of physicians to members in 1908, the American
Medical Association watched approvingly and linked this matter with
the low-pay issue. While it looked upon the pattern of lodge practice

as "pernicious and harmful," it added, "So long as the physician is paid a proper price for his services, such as will enable him to give his patients the care and attention to which they are entitled, there is no reason, either ethically or legally, why an agreement should not be made with an organization the same as with an individual."[22] To reduce the ruinous effect of competitive bidding it even suggested that fraternal orders give an examination to select the most suitable contract physician.

In tolerating a distasteful system, proponents of reform in contract practice brought up the argument they would use with telling effect in later decades about the danger of the "middleman." Early in the twentieth century the middleman symbolized such organizations as fraternal orders; later it would be government when the threat of state-administered health insurance appeared. Supposedly, the middleman often stood between the physician and the patient, preventing the delivery of proper medical care by the physician and proper payment by the patient.

At the Harrisburg session of the Pennsylvania Medical Association in 1911, Horace M. Alleman complained that "the physician is being exploited for the benefit of the middleman; his services are purchased at wholesale and sold at retail." Earlier Rexwald Brown, a physician of Santa Barbara, California, objected to contract practice with fraternal orders because the physician lost his dignity as he worked in constant fear of censure by the lodge.[23] In 1913 the contract practice committee of the California society declared that "the formation of societies for mutual benefit or insurance we do not condemn; but, whatever plan is adopted by such institutions the fee given the physician must be an individual affair between patient and doctor."[24] Clearly the committee implied that the medical profession should determine the payment scale in any plan. Though it left in doubt the question of whether a physician could accept contract practice under a schedule not of the profession's making, a few local societies answered emphatically, drafting resolutions forbidding their members from engaging in any contract practice below the minimum fee schedule.[25]

While societies hoping to reform contract practice sought professional controls to ensure greater remuneration, free choice of physician, and elimination of interference from the middleman, the California state organization pressed still another demand. It sought con-

trol over the recruitment policies of fraternal orders that would prevent their inclusion of families able to provide for medical care
through conventional means. At the annual session of 1912 the House
of Delegates adopted a resolution requiring members of the state
society to reject all contract work with fraternal orders or other organizations offering coverage based on per capita assessments of heads
of families with monthly incomes of $75 or more. Physicians accept-
ing such work faced the threat of expulsion from the local and state
societies.[26]

As many medical societies struggled with the reform problems of
contract practice the American Medical Association gave greater
attention to the issue. In 1911 it offered simple criteria for testing the
legitimacy of any contract plan. These criteria dealt with the economic justification of the contract, the possibility that it would harm
someone, and the possibility that the profession would be exploited
by middlemen. It found no justification for the contract practice of
fraternal orders, contending that in conducting these schemes they
exploited the profession and departed from the proper function of a
lodge. Actually, the *Journal* did little more than express opposition to
a form of contract practice that a portion of the profession tolerated
and hoped to improve.[27]

Not until two years later did the American Medical Association
move from a position of reluctant tolerance of fraternal schemes to
acceptance of their role in the provision of medical care. As the AMA
veered on a new course its Judicial Council led the way. In its historic
report to the Minneapolis session of the House of Delegates in 1913
the council surveyed the economic plight of the working classes, noting that 75 percent of American adult males had incomes of less than
$600 a year. It maintained that fraternal plans offered a form of insur-
ance against medical expense for many workmen who could lay up
no reserves against the cost of illness. "There is a point," it insisted,
"at which the ratio of fixed charges to total income is such that these
fraternal societies do become an economic necessity in the sense of
health insurance." As such, it concluded, they "must be accepted and
controlled, not condemned and shunned."[28]

Having called for the acceptance of fraternal contract practice plans
in a report adopted by the House of Delegates, the council called
upon the AMA to specify the upper limits of their usefulness. It

pressed the matter as one of greatest urgency, declaring that "the question comes down then to the designation of the weekly or monthly income at which this should be treated as an economic necessity and above which it is an economic luxury." Evading the issue of income limitation raised by the council, the delegates passed a resolution urging local societies to find ways to improve contract practice.[29]

The reforms medical societies sought to introduce in contract practice reached beyond their efforts to control the promotional schemes of fraternal orders. Their limited efforts also extended to hospital plans that developed largely unrestrained in the Progressive Era. The contract practice movement among hospitals, dating from the 1890s, passed from a stage of relative innocence early in the twentieth century to maturity when hospital associations became promotional agencies attempting to provide larger segments of the population with contract coverage. In combating these efforts the California society again pioneered in formulating policies to guide the profession in controlling contract practice.[30]

Los Angeles emerged as a center of strife when hospital associations joined with local hospitals in contractual schemes that exploited physicians. Promoters prospered from the contracts, hospitals added stability to their incomes, and physicians received in compensation little or nothing. But the interference of the middleman caused the formulation of policies defining the relationship between hospitals and physicians that stands out as a landmark for professional achievement in the Progressive Era.[31]

Drafting a code that the state organization soon adopted, the Los Angeles County Medical Society refused to allow the visiting staff to receive any compensation from the hospital or to allow the hospital to interfere in any way with the financial arrangement made between staff members and patients. No member of the society could render medical service to a member of a hospital association that offered coverage at a per capita fee to heads of families earning $75 or more a month. No hospital could maintain an outside dispensary in which it employed its resident staff, nor could it prevent the resident staff from accepting outside calls for service, nor interfere in the financial negotiations between the physician and patient. The code called for the appointment of a hospital commission that would grade hospitals on the observance of these rules as either approved or not approved.[32]

GRADUAL EXTINCTION POLICY

While some societies struggled to contain contract practice in narrow limits and others attempted to reform the system as it expanded, a less aggressive but vocal group made moderate suggestions anticipating its ultimate extinction. Medical publications of the Progressive Era gave some notice to physicians who did not turn opposition to contract practice into a crusade, but who believed that persistent emphasis on the ethical standards of medicine eventually would destroy the system. And, too, they believed that as the profession succeeded in reducing competition by gaining control over medical education it would remove a principal cause of contract practice. This group was more concerned with reforming the profession than with reforming contract practice, believing that in raising the ethics of the former the latter gradually would disappear.

The founding of the American Society of Medical Economics in New York City in 1912 stands out as an effort to raise the ethics of the profession by giving sufficient emphasis to what its president, E. Eliot Harris, called "practical medical sociology." He believed that reform depended upon the profession's recognition that there had been "no organized direction of the economics of medicine" and upon its willingness to treat the subject as more than an "appendix" to the scientific proceedings of a medical society. This organization proposed to instruct physicians on their duties to the public and on the public's obligation to them, hoping to curb abuses of the profession and to raise its income. This sentiment for gradual extinction through educational methods found expression elsewhere. Joseph N. McCormack insisted that medical schools give proper emphasis to professional ethics, and as early as 1907 the state of Michigan appealed for the teaching of the economics of professional practice in the medical schools of the state.[33]

CALL FOR IMMEDIATE ABOLITION

A fourth and final group of societies opposed all but governmental forms of contract practice and reliance on gradualism to destroy the system. Believing that all but government practice was hopelessly corrupt, adherents to this view called for the hasty abolition of every other type. Specific abuses in contract schemes mattered little to the Committee on Contract Work of the society in Erie County, New York, when it charged that it made no difference whether contract plans "overpaid or underpaid" the profession, for the practice provided under all such plans was "unethical, unjust, and in every sense injurious to the profession in general." Nor did it spare surgeons who accepted railroad contracts, declaring that it could not move against "small offenders without attacking these polished violators of the ethical laws who are seemingly responsible for all the others."[34]

Among factors responsible for the growth of contract practice the Committee on Contract Work included professional jealousy, ignorance of medical ethics, physician surplus, commercialism, and the disorganized state of the profession. It found 320 members who agreed to oppose contract practice but reported that some 200 others made no such commitment. It urged the society to use its influence against any physician who renewed a contract, declaring that "we must do him as we have done the advertising quack . . . we must do more. We must use antagonistic measures if persuasion fails to convince him of his error."[35]

Not all physicians who sought the hasty destruction of contract practice called for such harsh treatment. Probably the strongest opponent of the practice in Wisconsin was William F. Zierath of Sheboygan. Contending in 1907 that "contract practice in every phase, as an institution, must be completely and absolutely abolished," he said, "it can be done and it must be done, and we must do it now." But the solution did not lie in the expulsion or ostracism of wayward physicians. Only a thoroughly organized profession could abolish the system by employing less drastic and more subtle measures which he did not designate.[36]

VARIATIONS OF RESPONSE

The response of medical societies to the contract practice issue varied greatly. Probably most societies, hardly touched by the question, took no action. Some required that physicians about to engage in contract practice submit the contract to the local medical society for approval. Others required no more than that the practice plan meet the minimum pay level of the fee schedule.[37] In 1907 the state association in Michigan called for the compilation and publication of what may be viewed as an honor roll of physicians in the state who refused to accept contract practice. Other societies demanded expulsion from their ranks of all who continued in such practice. Editors of the *Pennsylvania Medical Journal* and the *California State Journal of Medicine* urged this action on societies in their states.[38]

EVOLUTION OF POLICY

Medical societies in the Progressive Era had much to do with shaping the course and nature of contract practice. But, in turn, the struggle to control the multiplying number of contract schemes did much to shape the profession's policies as well. From the inchoate and conflicting economic views of the profession at the beginning of the Progressive Era came policies that gained much wider acceptance before it closed. General charges of exploitation gave way to a lengthening chronicle of specific abuses and to a clearer analysis of points at issue. Medical societies began more precisely to identify areas of professional exploitation and to prescribe specific measures of control. They called for a widening of patient freedom by raising the idea of choice of physician to the status of a major issue. They brought added sanctity to the physician-patient relationship by setting over this relationship the specter of the middleman. In venturing to prescribe the upward limits of contract practice, they marked out a course that a desperate profession would search for again in the years ahead.

CHAPTER NINE

SOCIAL INSURANCE AND THE MEDICAL PROFESSION

Voluntary forms of contract practice still were a growing threat when the spread of workmen's compensation legislation in the second decade of the new century held out before the medical profession the prospect of even greater dangers. Most physicians were astonished at the success of the workmen's compensation movement when it rallied, after the New York Court of Appeals declared the state's compulsory law of 1910 unconstitutional, to secure passage of similar legislation in twenty-two other states by the beginning of World War I. As early as 1893, John Graham Brooks, commissioner of the United States Department of Labor, raised some interest in workmen's compensation with the publication of a report on the German industrial accident insurance system, but physicians, like most other groups, remained largely unmoved by proposals to shift from the family to society the social costs of production.[1]

CASE FOR COMPENSATION

The success of the movement for workmen's compensation insurance partially lay in the dismal performance of private carriers in the field of industrial liability insurance. Reports by nine liability companies submitted to a New York investigating agency showed that they paid only one in eight of the 414,681 claims received between 1906 and 1908. Some fifty American and five foreign firms collected $22,440,000 in premiums for liability insurance in 1908, from which they extracted from 35 to 60 percent for taxes, high salaries, exorbitant commissions, and office maintenance; no more than 25 percent ever reached disabled workers. Upon a capital deposit of $250,000, one foreign company remitted more than $259,000 to its home office in 1906 and more than $442,000 two years later. American companies often paid dividends of from 10 to 60 percent, and occasionally even more, on actual stock investment. Such appalling corporate abuses provoked W. H. Allport of the Illinois Occupational Disease Commission to charge, in 1910, that no moral, ethical, or industrial reason existed for the sale of liability insurance on the terms imposed by private carriers.[2]

State legislatures might have shown infinite tolerance of such abuses had not industrial groups detected advantages for themselves in the enactment of compensation statutes. Gradually their escapes from accident liability had diminished as state legislation finally narrowed their immunities in the application of common law. Finding only precarious refuge in recourse to the "fellow servant," the "assumption of risks," and the "contributory negligence" doctrines, they had hopes of deriving from workmen's compensation legislation an immunity that they could not otherwise secure. Furthermore, they could translate indefinite risks into a calculable expense that could be added to the costs of production.[3] Industrial interests eagerly joined a few labor spokesmen and a number of disinterested and public-spirited social groups in an uncomfortable alliance supporting the enactment of compensation laws.

Some public support for state-administered accident indemnity insurance systems followed publication of surveys depicting the human wreckage cast off by the industrial order and the absence or inadequacy of compensation awards. A major study in Allegheny County, Pennsylvania, of 235 cases of industrial fatalities among married men killed in the year following July 1906 showed that fifty-nine families received no compensation; sixty-five not more than $100; and for forty more the amount did not exceed $500. An investigation of seventy-four industrial deaths in New York City in 1908 showed that in 43 percent of the cases families of the victims received no compensation and in 41 percent less than $500.[4] Annual reports of the appalling death and injury rates among employees in the railroad and mining industries and the uncertain and inadequate settlement of liability claims shocked increasing numbers of Americans and much of the Western world.

PROFESSIONAL PASSIVITY

The medical profession did not share in the enthusiasm generated by the triumph of the movement for compensation. Medical spokesmen never forgot that they had been virtually excluded from panels drafting the statutes. Charging that "the rights of the medical profession were neither carefully considered nor conserved in most of the legislation," Francis D. Donoghue, medical adviser to the Industrial Accident Board of Massachusetts, remarked that physicians followed a generous course when "they were not early upon the legislative scene asking for their pound of flesh before carrying out the broad humanitarian principles" behind the legislation. Early in 1916 the editor of the *Wisconsin Medical Journal* observed that one-half of the states had enacted compensation laws and lamented that "in the creation of these laws the medical profession played practically no part. Its attitude was one of mere acquiescence."[5]

GROUNDS OF PROTEST

The profession's passivity in the struggle for compensation statutes differed sharply from its protests over the administration of the measures. Quickly it detected in the laws and their administration abuses it believed undermined the economic and ethical foundations of medical practice. Medical spokesmen raised three principal complaints against the spreading compensation system. Workmen's compensation laws, they charged, frequently denied the injured free choice of physicians; they disrupted the physician-patient relationship by injecting intermediate agents; and they required medical practice on intolerable financial terms. In the month California's law became effective (January 1914), Philip Mills Jones, the fiery editor of the *California State Journal of Medicine*, warned that insurance carriers already were organizing staffs of physicians and would deny injured workmen recourse to their own physicians. A month later he explained that when the employer had insurance the choice of physician passed to the insurance companies and that the patient had no choice. In June the state society attempted to adjust the free-choice principle to the demands of the legislation. It resolved that the *company insuring the employer* must have the right to select doctors from the association's entire membership. Burton R. Corbus, a Grand Rapids physician, had predicted that the free-choice principle would be sacrificed in Michigan to the compensation system.[6] Reports from other areas soon confirmed fears that compensation laws had instituted a form of contract practice that jeopardized the free-choice ethic. Anxiety over the issue did not subside. Only a few weeks after the United States entered

World War I, a troubled committee of the California society reported on violations of the free-choice principle in the administration of the state law and denounced all contract practice as unethical.[7]

Workmen's compensation laws soon awakened the profession to still another danger—they had forced the intrusion of intermediate parties into the physician-patient relationship. In private forms of contract practice the profession long had protested the presence of a third party, a lay organization that bargained for physicians' services. In workmen's compensation schemes it found three intermediate parties and sometimes four. The state, the employer, the insurance carrier, and, occasionally, agencies retailing physicians' services became involved in the provision of medical care. Because such innovations had legal sanction they appeared all the more dangerous and led the profession, for the first time, to question its confidence in the beneficence of the state.

The medical profession did not deny the necessity of state involvement in the compensation systems, but professional spokesmen charged that employers and the state had combined in a scheme that degraded medical practice. They showed that compensation laws confined the responsibility of employers for providing medical care to extremely limited periods. Among the first twenty-three states that enacted laws, one required payment of medical service for only one week, five for two weeks, three for ninety days, six only when a patient died without dependents, while two made no provision for medical payments. Representatives of the profession protested that the states, in absolving employers of responsibility for payment beyond brief periods, jeopardized the physician-patient relationship and often obstructed the delivery of adequate medical services. Furthermore, they showed that after employers secured immunity from liability suits under compensation laws, malpractice suits against physicians multiplied and that employers, in securing special exemptions, had joined with the state in releasing forces that terrorized the profession.[8]

The profession launched an even stronger attack on insurance carriers and independent agencies bargaining for physicians' services. Medical spokesmen knew all too well that insurance companies often had become the principal beneficiaries of the compensation programs. Charles H. Crounhart, retiring chairman of the Wisconsin Industrial Commission, informed the state medical association in 1915 that in the year ending 31 December 1914 compensation cost employers of Wisconsin over $2.2 million, that workmen or their dependents received only about $800,000 in cash benefits, that hospitals and doctors got only $400,000, while insurance carriers appropriated $1 million for administrative costs and profits. He also showed that insurance companies often forced their own fee schedules on the profession, established combined contracts with physicians and hospitals, and sometimes employed physicians on a salary basis.[9]

As the California law became effective, the editor of the state society's journal warned that physicians would be "squeezed" by insurance companies in the scramble for profits. Events quickly bore out his prediction. Only about two months later, councilors of the Los Angeles County Medical Association condemned the low and arbitrary fee schedule imposed by the California Casualty Insurance Board. It also opposed payment of physicians by the insurance board or by the state industrial commission "through any intermediate corporation or association seeking to make a profit for commercializing these services" and "sub-letting" them either "to insurance companies or other bodies." Nor would the councilors allow members to perform medical service for "secondary commercial associations" aiding in casualty cases at less than the fee schedule of the Los Angeles County Medical Association. The editor of Northwest Medicine reported in May 1912 that hospital associations in Washington had attempted to secure compensation cases and warned that any profit from this work would go to promoters who were not physicians.[10]

Compensation cases not only introduced problems peculiarly related to intermediate agencies but what the profession viewed as intolerable economic abuses as well. Medical leaders often protested that the low fee schedules drafted by insurance carriers or state industrial commissions usually fell below customary charges. The editor of the Journal of the Michigan State Medical Society contended that "not one of us" would agree to accept $30 for a herniotomy with an allowance of $1.50 each for perhaps ten visits. "This is not considered a reasonable fee from a private patient," he insisted, "and why should we discriminate between them and insurance corporations?"[11] The councilors of the Los Angeles county society urged the state industrial board to make clear that its fee schedule did not reflect standard fees but rather the limitations of the insurance fund and the low incomes of the insured. The Workmen's Compensation Commission of the New York state society attempted to make the system more palatable to members of the association when it insisted that compensation schedules did not replace county fee bills and applied only to the job-connected injuries of industrial employees. Societies often feared that compensation schedules would become standard charges and knew that somehow such schedules became public knowledge.[12]

But the profession knew that any fee schedule presented serious difficulties. The New York medical association even abandoned its own schedule as unworkable after state authorities had accepted it for the compensation system. Fee schedules binding members of local societies set *minimum* fees, but medical leaders realized that when schedules were drafted by government agencies and insurance companies the established fee became the maximum. They objected to any inelastic fee schedule since inflexible scales took no account of the varying complexities of treatment for similar disabilities. The editor of the *Journal of the Michigan State Medical Society* expressed the attitude of most physicians when he contended, "We are not working by the job or on piece work but expect, and rightly so, a reasonable and fair remuneration for the service we render in every individual instance."[13]

Physicians raised several other complaints against the compensation laws. The statutes, they charged, took no account of varying skills among physicians, rewarding the professional novice and the experienced physician alike. They complained that compensation laws frequently demanded work of physicians for which they got no remuneration. A physician from Washington charged that "in every report we are called on to give an opinion and a diagnosis, something that insurance companies pay us for, recognizing it as our means of livelihood, but this insurance company conducted by the state, assumes the right to demand these things without compensation." Furthermore, they found that compensation laws sometimes required the disclosure under oath of information long recognized by law and custom as "privileged communications," threatening the confidential relationship they considered essential to professional practice.[14]

AMERICAN ASSOCIATION FOR LABOR LEGISLATION

Whatever their complaints, physicians saw that their protests did not obstruct the progress of the workmen's compensation movement. In fact, they discovered that advocates of compensation laws often looked upon their enactment as but the opening victory in a long social insurance struggle. They also found that leadership of the social insurance forces came not from the ranks of industry or labor but increasingly from an enthusiastic and ideological organization of recent origin that boldly announced its goals and strategy. While medical spokesmen lamented that they had been ignored in the drafting of compensation statutes they received appeals from leaders of the American Association for Labor Legislation (AALL) seeking their assistance in a campaign for compulsory health insurance which they considered the "next great step in social legislation."[15]

Organized in New York City, 15 February 1906, as the sixteenth section of the International Association for Labor Legislation, the AALL had scored several victories for industrial workers and established an organ to deal with labor issues before launching its compulsory health insurance crusade. Under the brilliant leadership of the young labor economist John B. Andrews, who became the association's secretary and a member of its executive committee in 1909, the American Association for Labor Legislation secured enactment two years later of the first compulsory state law for reporting industrial diseases and shared in the work that led to the passage of the first workmen's compensation statutes. In January 1911 it launched the *American Labor Legislation Review*, which for its judicious and enlightened treatment of labor issues had no match among specialized publications concerned with social problems.[16]

COMPULSORY HEALTH INSURANCE ISSUE

American states seemed about ready to respond to the major challenges of industrialism when, in 1913, the AALL turned the attention of its social insurance committee from the subject of workmen's compensation to that of health insurance. Since thirteen states had adopted general compulsory laws after the invalidation of the New York Statute in 1910, the association believed it could carry compulsory health insurance through on a second wave of reform. At Chicago, in June 1913, it held its first conference on social legislation; another at the nation's capital in December devoted an entire section to health insurance. Isaac M. Rubinow, a physician, statistician, and member of the Social Insurance Committee, reflected the optimism of the Chicago conference when he compared the advance of workmen's compensation legislation with the rejection of the accident insurance principle by the "press, chair and bar" only five years before. But he deplored the "backwardness" of the nation's social thought and reminded the conference that the United States lagged a quarter of a century behind advanced European nations in dealing with the economic hazards of sickness.[17]

The American Association for Labor Legislation had other reasons for expecting the early enactment of health insurance laws. A decade and a half of inflation had practically nullified the income gains of workers across a broad economic spectrum, leaving them as helpless as ever in meeting the mounting cost of illness. The association knew that industrial insurance companies, gorged with profits, had made no real effort to offer family protection in medical crises, preferring to mete out paltry benefits at extortionate costs to unfortunate victims of their sickness insurance swindles.[18] Recent political developments convinced the AALL that compulsory health insurance would receive wide support among the working classes. They had shown interest in the establishment of the British National Health Insurance System and accounted for a good portion of the voters (28 percent) who had supported the Progressive party in 1912, which included in its platform a plank on social insurance written by Rubinow.[19] Furthermore, the AALL knew that health insurance rested on several principles already familiar to some Americans. A few industries, unions, and mutual benefit associations had adopted compulsory group insurance plans financed by employer and employee assessments. For several years the University of California had operated a prepaid student health care program, and as far back as 1798 the federal government had established a compulsory health insurance plan for sailors in the merchant marine.[20]

AALL'S CRUSADE BEGINS

Despite the familiarity of some Americans with health insurance principles, the AALL did not expect the public to accept hastily any compulsory health insurance plan. It prepared to educate influential groups on social insurance issues before launching a major political offensive. In an interim lasting from the establishment of its Social Insurance Committee early in 1913 through 1915 it undertook four major tasks: to bring into service its ablest health insurance spokesmen; to find support for health insurance among uncommitted groups and organizations; to take responsibility for drafting a model health insurance bill that might secure approval from health insurance groups, uncommitted organizations, and state legislatures;[21] and to plan periodic conferences to sustain interest in the movement.

Seldom has an organization put before the American public such able leadership. Through articles, editorials, books, addresses, and extensive correspondence, John B. Andrews set forth the challenges of industrialism and the urgency of compulsory health insurance while coordinating the work of the AALL. The outstanding authority on the American labor movement, John R. Commons, with whom Andrews coauthored a labor text in 1916, made frequent addresses on the health insurance issue. Rubinow, who published his classic study *Social Insurance* in 1913, gave unsparingly of his time to the movement. Other eminent scholars offering valuable assistance included John R. Seager and Joseph P. Chamberlain of Columbia University and Irving Fisher of Yale.[22]

APPEAL TO THE PROFESSION

The AALL sought support for health insurance from many groups, but expended its greatest effort on the medical profession. Since the profession had been largely ignored in the drafting of compensation legislation and was alienated by its operation, prospects for its support seemed unlikely at first. Yet the AALL found some medical leaders who favored the proposal and believed that it could overcome any general resistance by an extended period of persuasion. Even before its own interests had turned primarily to health insurance, scattered voices within the profession had deplored the dominance of individualistic fee-for-service practice, and within the profession organizations had formed to stress the social and economic aspects of medical service. Addressing the American Academy of Medicine in 1909, Wood Hutchison called the American system of practice "a makeshift and an anomaly," and three years later a prominent Brooklyn doctor, James P. Warbasse, charged that the physician, who should be a public servant, had become "a private tradesman engaged in a competitive business for a profit." As early as 1901 three southern state societies established a Committee on Sociological Science and the American Society of Medical Economics had been formed.[23]

The AALL made its first important effort to reach the profession near the opening of World War I. Growing international tensions did not dampen its ardor as several prominent physicians responded favorably to the health insurance appeal. In April 1914, Fitch C. E. Matti-

son, president of the California society, told delegates at the annual
session that the costs of industrial production should include expenses
attributable to accidents, sickness, and death. Industries, he said, that
insured their properties should raise no objection to health insurance
for their workers. He predicted a day when families would secure
adequate medical care without being pauperized in the process.[24]

Pressing the issue upon the profession, the AALL published its tentative standards for health insurance in the month the war began and
three months later made what appears to have been its first attempt
to carry the case for health insurance to a state society. In October, at
Oshkosh, John R. Commons spoke on "Social Insurance and the Medical Profession" before the Wisconsin medical association at a session
in which a physician from Sheboygen, William F. Zierath, made an
impassioned plea for a comprehensive national system of medical
care. The president, Charles S. Sheldon of Madison, showed his
approval of the health insurance principle when he told the session
that "some form of health insurance for the poor people has become
an economic necessity." In the same month Rubinow presented the
AALL's case for health insurance in an address to the Association of
Physicians of Long Island, which the American Medical Association
published three months later in the *Journal* and circulated as a
reprint.[25]

When the AALL planned in 1915 to make health insurance a political issue the following year, it sought a positive reaction from physicians. As it had hoped, favorable journalistic comments on the subject came from some outstanding medical editors including Philip
Mills Jones, who was both the editor of the California journal and a
trustee of the AMA.[26] From several prominent physicians it secured
assistance in drafting the tentative health insurance bill, which it
circulated among interested medical and lay groups in November for
further criticism and revision. Its work led the AMA late in the year
to create its own social insurance committee headed by Alexander
Lambert, a prominent health insurance advocate, who soon secured
the services of Rubinow as the committee's secretary.[27]

LEAGUE WITH LAYMEN

Other developments convinced the AALL that it need not wait
much longer to test the political strength of the issue. The Industrial
Relations Commission, which had spent three years investigating the
problems of labor and management, submitted its final report in 1915,

recommending a system of compulsory health insurance.[28] Governor Hiram Johnson of California had just become the first to appoint a committee on social insurance to study the issue. Furthermore, the Progressive National Service, created by leaders of the Progressive party to perpetuate its principles, began to show greater interest in health insurance. Even the Metropolitan Life Insurance Company seemed to feel the growing threat of health insurance agitation when it conducted investigations of major illnesses in several American cities beginning with Rochester, New York, and Trenton, New Jersey, in the fall of 1915.[29]

TURN TO POLITICS

The AALL and the AMA presented a united front as the health insurance movement entered its political phase in January 1916. Not only did the two organizations work in close contact, but two members of the AALL's social insurance committee held positions with the same committee of the AMA. Largely through Alexander Lambert, who served on both committees and as chairman of the AMA's Judicial Council, the organizations combined their strength. Contacts between the AALL and the AMA indicated the unity they had achieved. On 6 January, Lambert sent Andrews a list of members of the AMA's Judicial Council and Council on Health and Public Instruction to whom he could send publications of his organization. As the AALL got the model bill before the legislatures of New York, Massachusetts, and New Jersey, it called upon officers of the AMA for further criticisms. On 7 January, Andrew's assistant, Olga S. Halsey, wrote to Alexander R. Craig, secretary of the AMA, for his suggestions, declaring that the AALL had no intention of drafting the medical sections in final form without the cooperation of the medical profession. On 18 January, Andrews advised Irving Fisher that Frederick R. Green, chairman of the AMA's Council on Health and Public Instruction, would be in New York two days later to consult with them on the health insurance issue. The next day he sent Lambert a copy of the medical sections of the British health insurance act and the Fabian report on its operation.[30]

THE MODEL BILL

Negotiations between the AALL and the AMA early in 1916 brought about two additional drafts of the bill before the measure became nearly final. Adhering to the principle that low-income groups should be protected against the economic hazards of illness while higher income classes should be exempted from compulsory coverage, it called for inclusion of manual workers and some other low-income employees with annual incomes of $1,200 or less and for their dependents. Benefits ranged from medical, surgical, nursing, hospital care, and the provision of medical supplies to payments for income loss in sickness equal to two-thirds of an employee's wages for a maximum of twenty-six weeks in any one year and funeral benefits not exceeding fifty dollars. The bill placed two-fifths of the cost of the program on employers, two-fifths on employees, and one-fifth on the state.

The measure contained flexible organizational and administrative features hopefully designed to reduce the medical profession's suspicion of standardized service and to meet diverse sectional needs. To be administered by a state social insurance commission in consultation with advisory boards appointed by state medical societies, the proposed system provided for three administrative approaches. It allowed employment of a panel of physicians, use of salaried physicians, and restriction of physicians' services to specified geographical areas. The panel system offered membership to all legally qualified physicians, provided for free choice among panel physicians, and imposed limitations on the number of patients any physician could treat.[31]

The model bill prescribed no single precise method for remunerating physicians, but offered several alternatives. Lambert explained that adequate remuneration even within a system guaranteeing 100 percent collections raised difficult questions. He cited the disadvantages of the capitation fee and the high cost of payment by visit; he suggested a combination of the two plans, or perhaps employment of physicians on a salaried basis that had proved successful among railroads. The AALL not only allowed for flexibility in the measure's payment features, but showed additional capacity for concession when, apparently to reduce political resistance to a comprehensive bill, it removed family coverage from the drafts introduced into the Massachusetts and New York legislatures allowing benefits to low-income wage earners only.[32]

MOVEMENT GAINS MOMENTUM

The feverish activities of the AALL and the AMA gave the health insurance movement remarkable momentum in the spring of 1916. In

April the editor of the *New England Medical Gazette* responded to Andrews's request that he publicize the measure with an extensive and favorable treatment, and before the month had passed Athel C. Burnham of New York gave a favorable analysis of the bill in the *Medical Record*. On 3 April, John B. McAlister, president of the Pennsylvania state association, presented the advantages of health insurance to physicians of the society of Harrisburg and Dauphin County and secured their support of the bill then in the state legislature. On 19 April, Rubinow read a paper on "Health Insurance in Relation to the Public Dispensary" at a meeting of officials from the outpatient clinics of New York City, which received wide publicity when the AMA's Council on Health and Public Instruction circulated it as the third pamphlet in its Social Insurance Series.[33]

Even more favorable prospects for the success of the health insurance movement appeared in May. Andrews won cautious support from George Blumer, dean of the Yale Medical School, whose favorable article on the issue appeared in the *Pennsylvania Medical Journal* and the *Proceedings of the Connecticut State Medical Society*. A more notable victory came when a conference of state and territorial health officers and representatives from the United States Public Health Service endorsed a report favorable to health insurance prepared by a committee headed by William C. Woodward, who also directed the AMA's Committee on Medical Legislation.[34] Furthermore, Andrews got an opportunity to explain the bill before the annual meeting of the National Association for the Study and Prevention of Tuberculosis and to employ the language of Royal Meeker, United States commissioner of labor statistics, in replying to charges that health insurance would make a "spoonfed mollycoddle" of the independent citizen. Like Meeker, he conceded that such would be a "cruel calamity," but preferred "a race of sturdy, contented, healthful mollycoddles" to "the most ferociously independent and self-reliant super-race of tubercular, rheumatic and malarial cripples tottering unsocialistically along the socialized highways" toward a "socialized or mutualized graveyard full of little individualistic slabs erected to the memory of the independent and self-reliant dead."[35]

Untiring in his effort to build support among professional leaders, Andrews mailed a form letter to sixty-six editors of medical journals on 19 May explaining the progress of the movement. Declaring that the AALL had secured the introduction of bills into the legislatures of Massachusetts, New York, and New Jersey, he announced that California already had appointed a commission to study the issue and that Congress and the legislature of Massachusetts contemplated similar action.[36] A week later Rubinow reflected Andrews's confidence when he told a meeting of the Casualty, Actuarial and Statistical Society of America, "The [social insurance] movement must go on, not because there are a few 'social workers' who advocate it, but because there exists the spirit of the new American democracy which will not permit the fear and anguish of destitution to stare in the face of millions of our citizens forever, and because the insurance method has been recognized as an effective weapon to combat it."[37] No group, however, seemed more receptive to Rubinow's appeal than physicians. After he spoke before the AMA's section of Preventive Medicine and Public Health at the Detroit session in June 1916, the association published his paper in the journal and circulated it as a reprint.[38]

Favorable responses from the state medical societies of Michigan, Wisconsin, and California encouraged the health insurance advocates during the summer and early fall. In July 1916 the editor of the *Journal of the Michigan State Medical Society* published the tentative model bill, writing strongly in its defense, and in October the Wisconsin Medical Society at its annual session endorsed the health insurance principle.[39] In California, where a committee chosen by the state society explored the issue with a committee appointed by the governor, prospects for the early enactment of a health insurance law appeared brightest. Philip Mills Jones, as editor of the *California State Journal of Medicine,* ran favorable reports on health insurance, and by September, Rubinow had widened support for the movement by filling twenty-five speaking engagements throughout the state in ninety days.[40]

The movement in California brought forth other talented and persuasive spokesmen. Among lesser leaders the most impressive was James L. Whitney, whose case for health insurance presented to the San Francisco Medical Society on 12 September was highly persuasive and logical. Stressing the advantages of health insurance in areas of preventive medicine, he showed that the fee-for-service system often denied patients the advantage of professional consultations that would detect illnesses in early stages and frequently deprived physicians of opportunities to provide extended and effective treatment. Convinced that the fee-for-service system had largely outlasted its usefulness, he asked, "Is it necessary that a doctor should be paid by the piece to induce him to do honest work? Are physicians the only men in the world who cannot be trusted to receive a salary and deliver full value for it?"[41]

The December meeting of the AALL in Columbus in 1916 served as a fitting climax of an eventful year. The American Institute of Homeopathy only recently had endorsed the principle of health insurance, and at Columbus prominent leaders of the regular profession announced or reaffirmed their support. Frank Billings of Chicago, a prominent medical educator, who served twice as president of the AMA and later as a trustee, declared that he "unequivocally" favored compulsory health insurance, and C. D. Selby, secretary-treasurer of the Ohio State Medical Association announced his support.[42] Frederick R. Green, secretary of the AMA's Council on Health and Public Instruction, revealed his own view when he said, "While it is probably true that a large per cent of the profession would to-day vote against the proposition, I do not believe that there is a single member of the medical profession who has given it careful and at all exhaustive study who is against it."[43] Alexander Lambert reaffirmed his strong support of health insurance, and Irving Fisher, a Yale University economist, indicated that the profession might lead the movement when he observed that the state societies in Pennsylvania and Wisconsin already had endorsed the insurance principle. Andrews, who had just begun to circulate a new pamphlet among physicians containing the latest version of the model bill, shared this hope and had an even greater reason for optimism when the last issue of the AMA's *Journal* in 1916 published the new medical features of the bill and called upon physicians to offer criticisms and suggestions.[44]

CREST OF THE CRUSADE

The early weeks of 1917 raised enthusiasm among health insurance advocates to its crest. On 25 January, after extensive investigation, California's social insurance commission reported that "health insurance of the wage earners would seem a tremendous step forward in social progress," and on 12 February, after holding fourteen public hearings and thirty-two executive sessions, the Massachusetts commission announced its unanimous acceptance of the insurance principle. Although recommending further study before final enactment of a program, it suggested a system wide enough "to safeguard every wage earner in the Commonwealth from certain of the evils of sickness, unemployment and old age."[45] Two days later New Jersey's Commission on Old Age, Insurance and Pensions decided to prepare a health insurance bill for introduction into the legislature, and less than two weeks after the United States entered World War I the Connecticut legislature established a commission to study the issue. Early in 1917, Senator William E. Borah of Idaho expressed his approval of health insurance while Governors Samuel W. McCall (Massachusetts), Emmet W. Boyle (Nevada), and Hiram W. Johnson and William D. Stephens (both of California), recommended it to the legislatures of their respective states. Governor Emanuel L. Philipp (Wisconsin) called for a commission to study its merits, and Governor Henry W. Keyes (New Hampshire) spoke favorably of the health insurance proposal.[46]

Powerful medical journals also appeared to have been deeply impressed by the movement, and prominent professional leaders continued their crusade. Late in January the *Journal of the American Medical Association* emphasized "that the time for the medical profession to interest itself in social insurance legislation is now, while legislation is in a formatve stage." In the same issue, Alexander Lambert charged that "self-respecting people of small means" could not secure the medical services they needed under prevailing conditions and that illness among the poor often brought destitution.[47] The following month the *New York State Journal of Medicine* published Irving Fisher's plea for health insurance made before the Medical Society of the County of New York. And while these medical journals and spokesmen cited the merits of health insurance, Rubinow traveled twenty-five thousand miles in the first half of the year carrying the crusade to professional and lay audiences in strategic areas of the nation.[48]

CRUSADE IN CRISIS

Exuberant over favorable responses to the insurance issue, health insurance advocates took too lightly the opposition their crusade aroused. Moving through flurries of dissent early in 1916, they faced the headwinds before the year had closed. Choosing New York as the first state in which to test the issue (and with no expectation of immediate victory), they secured introduction of the Mills bill on 24 January. On 26 February, Eden V. Delphey, chairman of the Health

Insurance Committee of the Federation of Medical Economic Leagues, voiced his opposition to several features of the measure and asked Andrews to see that the bill guaranteed free choice of physicians, compulsory panel membership of all physicians working under the system, and adequate representation of physicians on administrative boards. Two days later the Medical Society of the County of New York went further and summarily rejected the bill.[49] At senate hearings in March, James R. Rooney, chairman of the Committee of Five appointed by the Medical Society of the State of New York to deal with the issue, opposed the measure, while Samuel J. Kopetzsky, chairman of the Committee on Legislation of the Medical Society of the County of New York, called it "untimely" and said it would legalize the "worst evils of contract practice." When Alexander Lambert testified for the bill on 16 March, Andrews's assistant commended his action, believing that it counteracted much of the "rather disagreeable opposition of some of the doctors." Despite conferences in April between representatives of the AALL and societies of the state and county of New York, opposition among physicians persisted, even preventing passage of a bill that Senator Odgen Mills introduced on 29 March, proposing establishment of a commission to study the insurance issue.[50]

Proponents of health insurance overcame opposition to a bill establishing an investigatory commission in Massachusetts but met growing attacks from health insurance foes in several states. Major insurance companies, finding their own interests endangered by health insurance agitation, tried successfully in many instances to convince doctors that their welfare too was threatened. Even spokesmen for some labor unions saw in health insurance the specter of government paternalism and spread fears among many workmen. Nor had hospital administrators united in support of such insurance, and they sometimes seemed easily swayed by arguments raised against it.[51]

When Emery R. Hayhurst, director of the Division of Industrial Hygiene of Ohio, appeared on a panel before the Ohio Hospital Association late in May 1916, he noted that a remark of a conferee charging that health insurance would bring on the "Germanizing" of medical care got the greatest applause. At the Conference on Social Insurance that year, Grant Hamilton, member of the legislative committee of the American Federation of Labor, declared that workers did not want "benevolently administered saving of pennies" and added, "Get off the backs of the workers, and there will be no need for insurance, for the wage earners, like employers, will have enough to live on and to provide for emergencies without 'aid.'" Before a section of the American Association for the Advancement of Science late in December, Edson S. Lott, president of the United States Casualty Company, traced health insurance back to Germany where, he believed, the state had, in effect, appropriated private property for public use.[52]

As the offensive against health insurance mounted late in 1916, the American Association for Labor Legislation suffered two crippling blows in rapid succession. On 27 November death claimed the courageous editor of the *California State Journal of Medicine*, Philip Mills Jones, who had vowed several months before to keep this periodical open to the advocates of health insurance. Jones expressed considerable sympathy for their cause, and had he lived, surely he would have exposed the propaganda against health insurance that soon poured in on doctors of this politically crucial state.[53]

The movement suffered a second shock when the bitterest and most outspoken enemy of health insurance came out of the ranks of the American Association of Labor Legislation itself. Frederick L. Hoffman, while serving as statistician of the Prudential Life Insurance Company, also held positions on the General Administrative Council and the Executive Committee of the AALL. Increasingly torn by his divided loyalties as the leadership of the AALL pressed for health insurance, he finally and formally severed connection with the association in December 1916 and turned at once into its fiercest and most effective critic.[54] In fact, his influence became so great among foes of health insurance that John R. Commons declared with little or no exaggeration nearly two years later that the literature against such insurance "all originates from one source; all of the ammunition, all of the facts and statistics that you may come across, no matter who gives them to you, will be found to go back to the Prudential Insurance Co. of America, and to Mr. Frederick L. Hoffman, their very eminent statistician."[55]

Commons spoke primarily of the use health insurance foes made of Hoffman's 101-page pamphlet, *Facts and Fallacies of Compulsory Health Insurance* which the Prudential Press of Newark, New Jersey, published in 1917. But months before this critique appeared he assailed health insurance and its proponents. At the Conference on Social Insurance in 1916 he deplored the "vast government organization, with inquisitorial and dictatorial powers" that a health insurance system allegedly would create and contended that neither representatives of labor nor of industry sought such a system.[56] He renewed his attack before the section on Social and Economic Science of the American Association for the Advancement of Science on 26 December, making charges that he soon incorporated into his widely circulated pamphlet. In this pamphlet, and very likely in the address, he referred to leaders of the AALL and to their alleged misrepresentations when he charged, "For recklessness in utterances, for broad allegations contrary to the facts, for fatuous reliance upon foreign experiences, the arguments in favor of compulsory health insurance have not their parallel in the whole history of social agitation and labor reform."[57]

Late in 1916 the principal opponents of health insurance increasingly allowed calm consideration of the insurance issue to give way to extravagant and temperamental outbursts. The brief period providing for a tolerant and judicious treatment of the issue had passed. Writing in November, Donald M. Gedge, a California physician, reflected the trend: "Already the burden of life has fallen upon the vast concourse of humans, comprising the so-called middle class, while misconceived sympathies are being extravagantly squandered upon the undeserving, wasteful and improvident. Herein lies the productive field for the Socialists, the reformers and so-called social workers." He added: "If we are to be reduced to the acceptance of a State-regulated remuneration, why not the plumber, the carpenter, or any other tradesman? I hold it as much a misfortune for my boiler in my kitchen to burst as that the patients' family be suddenly stricken with illness—yet the state makes no provision for the repair of my boiler, neither does it prescribe what the plumber shall be paid."[58]

As the new year opened, near panic spread among forces opposing compulsory health insurance. Insurance companies and their front organizations, a few national associations, several lawyers, and some outspoken doctors launched a major attack as several governors and legislative commissions endorsed the health insurance principle. Hoffman stood in the front ranks of the fight, but other spokesman of major insurance companies rallied to his side. On 22 January 1917 he told the National Civic Federation (whose legislative committee included Leo K. Frankel, third vice president of the Metropolitan Life Insurance Company) that health insurance would reduce medical practice to "an intolerable degree of inferiority" and that it was "no more or less than a skillfully disguised form of poor relief." A few days later he attempted to defend the public health record of the United States which the AALL had criticized by showing that the recent mortality statistics of Massachusetts compared favorably with those of Prussia.[59]

On 22 January, William Gale Curtis, presenting the view of the Insurance Economic Society of America, asked the Medical Society of the County of New York, "Can you imagine the horde of constables necessary to even try to enforce such a law—dashing from house to house weekly in pursuit of nickels and dimes, and failing to collect them, arresting the people?"[60] In February, Philemon Tecumseh Sherman (a New York City lawyer and son of the Civil War general) published a ninety-four-page tract charging with some truth that the model bill failed to provide medical aid to those who needed it most. But he also contended that only "the administrative efficiency, police organization and iron discipline of the German government" made its system "practicable and effective" and warned that Americans should not be swept away by the "propaganda of compulsion."[61]

On the medical front the AALL actually lost its chance to capture strategic salients. Cleverly exploiting the crises that pushed the United States into World War I, opponents of insurance made surprising headway among doctors as they identified a compulsory system with German regimentation. On 22 January, the Medical Society of the County of New York denounced the model bill Senator Mills had reintroduced in the state assembly.[62] The American Medical Association had taken no official stand on compulsory health insurance and carried a letter critical of Hoffman's proposal in its *Journal* of 10 February. Three days later the Chicago Medical Society adopted perhaps the bitterest documents attacking health insurance that any society had ever drafted, which was endorsed by the Health Insurance Committee of the Illinois Medical Society (see Appendix VII).[63] Support in California gave way in April when the San Diego session of the AMA largely ignored a cautious and fairly favorable report of its Committee on Compulsory Health Insurance and adopted instead a resolution offered by the Committee on New Business stating that "although such health insurance may quite possibly become highly desirable at some future day, for the present it is best to withhold legislation until such time as experience has proven the worth of social insurance as we now have it, and until political and economic affairs in our country have again become normal."[64]

By April 1917 the health insurance movement had received setbacks from which it never recovered. Yet gains its leaders reported early in the year, although somewhat illusory, brought the crusade to its climax. The strongest opposition came from the insurance companies both in the period before the United States entered World War I and in the abortive revival of the crusade that occurred soon after the conflict closed. Health insurance proponents never made concessions to insurance companies that might have tempered their opposition, retaining, for instance, funeral benefits in the model bill.[65] Critics of health insurance easily frightened physicians by their charge that the proposal would revive the worst evils of contract practice against which so many doctors had fought so long. The unfortunate experiences of many physicians with the operation of newly established workmen's compensation systems made them more receptive to the propaganda of insurance companies and more fearful of government controls.[66]

The health insurance movement provoked similar responses from other groups. The struggling armies of labor remained largely apathetic, and some of their leaders (including Samuel Gompers) were distinctly hostile. Industrial organizations, finding little in health insurance that advanced their interests, generally fought the movement. Furthermore, the philosophy of health insurance conflicted with some attitudes widely and deeply rooted in American thought. It challenged the adequacy of the principle of private paternalism in dealing effectively with most social ills. To many Americans it also appeared to encourage a drift toward prodigality and vice. In March 1917, Frank F. Dresser, a prominent Masschusetts lawyer and an authority on employer liability legislation, raised this aspect of the ethical issue. Among other reasons for his opposition to health insurance he included its coverage of illnesses that bore no direct relationship to employment and that arose as consequences of intemperate and wanton lives.[67] Finally, as health insurance advocates later realized, their movement had been unfortunately timed. It came too late to receive much momentum from the general reform spirit of the Progressive Era and too early to avoid the distracting impact of World War I.

CHAPTER TEN

SUMMARY

The Progressive Era marks the most fateful epoch in the history of the American medical profession. No period of comparable length broke more ties with the past while strengthening others or exercised so fateful an influence on the future. In this era for the first time the profession created a national political base, frequently attached as much or more importance to political means as to scientific ends, and developed a talented political leadership never matched before, or probably since, in American medical history. Through an alliance with the law it accomplished in less than two decades at the state level more than it had achieved politically since the states were formed. In reaching its goals it determined to project a more favorable public image, and in the process it surpassed all other pressure groups or business interests as a pioneer in public relations strategy. In no other era did medical organizations make greater attempts to cultivate a professional mystique while physicians increasingly took on the role of businessmen. No other era fixed so firmly the profession's social attitudes or dictated so completely its political course for decades ahead.

In general the medical profession shared the basic tenets and temperament of Progressivism. In the new century it reflected the optimism that Progressivism had inherited from the old and a confidence in American progress that even survived the shock of World War I. The Progressive insistence on the application of scientific techniques in dealing with some social problems was readily proclaimed in the field of medicine where dogmatism and empiricism had prevailed widely. In this era the profession largely cleared the scene of inferior regular medical schools and of institutions serving as fountainheads of sectarian chaos. In the belated and limited struggle with problems arising largely from urbanization and industrialization, it showed no hesitancy, until late in the Progressive Era, to employ the power of the state that it had used so effectively in putting its own house in order.

Just as conservative business interests shaped the form of Progressive legislation to reduce industrial risks and to diminish the hazards of competition, the medical profession fought much the same battle for limited competition strictly controlled. Like captains of finance and industry, who imposed their will on legislation to create regularity and predictability, medical leadership brought cohesion out of chaos, discipline out of division, and dictation out of dissent. It could all but ignore some issues threatening cohesion and depend upon the federal nature of the AMA to prevent their emergence as major problems. Just as Progressivism preserved the restrictions of color barriers and widened economic and political gaps between the races, medical societies also reflected provincial racial views.

Medical leadership of the Progressive Era attempted to elevate the ethics of the profession that had eroded in the commercialism of the Gilded Age. Substantial evidence indicates that it wrought a favorable and considerable change. But often (and in part as a result of Joseph N. McCormack's organizational crusade) it gave higher priority to medical etiquette than to medical ethics, leaving much of the profession largely ignorant of the latter. As medical leaders sought to reduce hostility and criticism among doctors, they unwittingly protected abuses that the profession usually would not control and that the public generally could not prevent. Physicians increasingly yielded to the imperatives of silence and found security in acquiescence when confronting the pressures of dominant professional thought. The trend toward specialization, making physicians ever more dependent on referrals, only increased tendencies toward conformity and conditioned accent.

Much of the mythology and mystery that has enshrouded the profession for many years diminishes in the light of the Progressive Era. In the depression decade physicians acquired the image of a persecuted and embattled group, recently drawn into politics, novices confronting the leviathan state. Actually, much of its leadership developed political expertise before World War I began and entered the New Deal as veterans of countless political struggles. The public has looked upon the profession's political success as a reflection of dogmatic and inflexible policies. Actually, the Progressive Era shows that the profession gained its political strength through deft and adroit politics and countless compromises. In still another way the profession projected, perhaps unwittingly, a less than faithful image. As it established patterns increasingly shifting the cost of medical training to the public, it made no effort to acknowledge social contributions to its advance or to qualify its insistence on rugged individualism and self-reliance. Furthermore, as it succeeded in perpetuating the ancient and priceless image of physicians as tireless, uncomplaining, and sacrificing servants, major developments of the period forced them increasingly into a less altruistic role.

But behind the profession's mastery of public relations in the Progressive Era lay its mounting contributions to crusades for reform. By the close of the Progressive period it had largely erased a tarnished public image that again haunts medical leadership as the last quarter of the twentieth century begins. The profession confronted public indifference and apathy as it launched its work in the first decade; it now confronts resentment and demand for drastic and effective crisis measures to meet growing medical problems. Medical spokesmen may disregard the constructive role of the profession in the Progressive Era and largely perpetuate its mistakes or they may recapture public confidence by offering the nation similar qualities of leadership again.

APPENDIXES

APPENDIX I. STANDARDS OF MEDICAL EDUCATION (Adopted by AMA, July 1905)

THE IDEAL STANDARD. The ideal standard to be aimed at from the present viewpoint should consist of: (a) Preliminary education sufficient to enable the candidate to enter our recognized universities. The passing upon such qualifications by the state authorities. (b) A five-year medical course, the first year of which should be devoted to physics, chemistry and biology, and such arrangements should be made that this year could be taken either in a school of liberal arts or in the medical school. Of the four years in pure medical work, the first two should be spent in laboratories of anatomy, physiology, pathology, pharmacology, and the last two in close contact with patients in dispensaries and hospitals in the study of medicine, surgery, obstetrics and the specialties. (c) A sixth year as an interne in a hospital or dispensary should then complete the medical course.

Under such a scheme the majority of men would begin the study of medicine between 18 and 19 years of age, and would graduate from the hospital interneship at from 24 to 25. A college education is recognized as a desirable preparation for limited numbers of men, but it is thought that it is not and never will be desirable to make such college education a requirement to the study of medicine, as it would make the age at graduation from 27 to 28 years, which is regarded as too late a period at which the young medical man should begin his life's work. It is obvious that this very desirable scheme of requirements can not be at once demanded or recommended.

STANDARD NOW RECOMMENDED. The standard of requirements now recommended prerequisite to the practice of medicine consists of five cardinal points, as follows:

1. Preliminary requirements to be a high school education or its equivalent, such as would admit the student to one of our recognized universities.

2. Preliminary requirements to be passed on by a state official, such as the superintendent of public instruction, and also by an official of the medical college.

3. A medical training in a medical college, having four years of not less than thirty weeks each year, of thirty hours per week of actual work.

4. Graduation from an approved medical college required to entitle the candidate to an examination before a state examining board.

5. The passing of a satisfactory examination before a state examining board.

Source: *JAMA* 47 (25 Aug. 1906): 627.

APPENDIX II. TEN POINT STANDARD OF MEDICAL SCHOOL INSPECTION

1. The success of the graduates of the school before the examination Boards.

2. Standards and enforcement of satisfactory preliminary educational entrance requirements.
3. The general character and extent of the college curriculum.
4. The medical school buildings.
5. Laboratory facilities and instruction.
6. Dispensary facilities and instruction.
7. Hospital facilities and instruction.
8. Extent to which the first two years are offered by men devoting their time to teaching and the evidences of original research.
9. Extent to which the school is conducted solely as an institution for teaching medicine rather than as a means for the profit of the faculty, directly or indirectly.
10. The owning of a library, museum, charts, models, etc.

Source: *JAMA* 48 (18 May 1907): 1702.

APPENDIX III. ESSENTIALS OF AN ACCEPTABLE MEDICAL COLLEGE

1. Strict enforcement of all standards and requirements, the college itself to be held responsible for any instances where they are not enforced.

2. A requirement for admission of at least a four-year high school education superimposed on eight years of grammar school work, or the actual equivalent education, this to consist of 14 units as defined by the College Entrance Examining Board and required by the Carnegie Foundation for the Advancement of Teaching.

3. As soon as conditions warrant, the minimum requirement for admission should be enlarged to include at least one year's college work each in physics, chemistry and biology and a reading knowledge of at least one modern language, preferably German or French.

4. A requirement that students be in actual attendance in the college within the first week of each annual session and thereafter.

5. That actual attendance at classes be insisted on except for good cause, such as for sickness, and that no credit be given under any circumstances for less than 80 per cent of attendance on each course.

6. That advanced standing be granted only to students of other acceptable colleges and that in granting advanced standing there shall be no discrimination against the college's full-course students.

7. Careful and intelligent supervision of the entire school by a dean or other executive officer who holds, and has sufficient authority to carry out, fair ideals of medical education as interpreted by modern demands.

8. A good system of records showing conveniently the credentials, attendance, grades and accounts of the student.

9. A fully graded course covering four years of at least 30 weeks, exclusive of holidays, and at least 30 hours per week of actual work: this course should be clearly set forth in a carefully prepared and printed schedule of lectures and classes.

10. Two years of work consisting largely of laboratory work in thoroughly equipped laboratories in anatomy, histology, embryology, physiology, chemistry (inorganic, organic and physiologic), bacteriology, pathology, pharmacology, therapeutics and clinical diagnosis.

11. Two years of clinical work largely in hospitals and dispensaries, with thorough courses in internal medicine (including physical diagnosis, pediatrics, nervous and mental diseases), surgery (including surgical anatomy and operative surgery on the cadaver), obstetrics, gynecology, laryngology, rhinology, ophthalmology, otology, dermatology, hygiene and medical jurisprudence.

12. At least six expert, thoroughly trained instructors in the laboratory branches, salaried so they may devote their time to instruction and to that research without which they cannot well keep up with rapid progress being made in their subjects. These instructors should rank sufficiently high to have some voice in the conduct of the college. There should also be a sufficient number of assistants in each department to look after the less important details.

13. The medical teaching should be of at least the same degree of excellence as obtains in our recognized liberal arts colleges and technical schools.

14. The members of the faculty, with a few allowable exceptions, should be graduates of institutions recognized as medical colleges and should have had a training in all departments of medicine. They should be appointed because of their ability as teachers and not because they happen to be on the attending staff of some hospital or for other like reasons.

15. The college should own or entirely control a hospital in order that students may come into close and extended contact with patients under the supervision of the attending staff. The hospital should have a sufficiently large number of patients to permit the student to see and study the common varieties of surgical and medical cases as well as a fair number in each of the so-called specialties.

16. The college should have easily accessible hospital facilities of not less than 200 patients which can be utilized for clinical teaching (for senior classes of 100 students or less), these patients to represent in fair proportion all departments of medicine.

17. The college should have additional hospital facilities for children's diseases, contagious diseases and nervous and mental diseases.

18. Facilities for at least five maternity cases for each senior student, who should have actual charge of these cases under the supervision of the attending physician.

19. Facilities for at least 30 autopsies during each college session (for senior classes of 100 students or less).

20. A dispensary, or out-patient department, under the control of the college, the attendance to be a daily average of 60 cases (for senior classes of 100 students or less), the patients to be carefully classified, good histories and records of the patients to be kept and the material to be well-used.

21. The college should have a working medical library to include the more modern text and reference books and 10 or more leading medical per-

iodicals: the library room to be easily accessible to students during all or the greatest part of the day: to have suitable tables and chairs and to have an attendant in charge.

22. A working medical museum having its various anatomic embryologic, pathologic and other specimens carefully prepared, labeled and indexed so that any specimen may be easily found and employed for teaching purposes.

23. A supply of such useful auxiliary apparatus as stereopticon, a reflectoscope, carefully prepared charts, embryologic or other models, manikins, dummies for use in bandaging, a Reontgen ray or other apparatus now so generally used in medical teaching.

24. The college should show evidences of reasonably modern methods in all departments and evidences that the equipment and facilities are being intelligently used in the training of medical students.

25. A statement in which the college's requirements for admission, tuition, time of attendance on the classes, sessions and graduation are clearly set forth should be given, together with complete lists of its matriculants and latest graduating class in regular annual catalogues or announcements.

Source: "Report of the Council on Medical Education," *JAMA* 54 (11 June 1910): 1974–75.

APPENDIX IV. STRUCTURE OF MEDICAL BOARDS, 1917

COMPOSITE BOARDS				SINGLE BOARDS	
4 Systems	3 Systems	2 Systems	Unspecified		
Ariz.	Ga.	Minn.	Kan.	Ala.	Wyo.
Ind.	Ida.	N.D.	Mass.	Calif.	Mont.
Ky.	Neb.	S.D.	Mo.	Colo.	N.H.
Mich.	Nev.		Ohio	Conn.	N.M.
Ore.	N.J.		Okla.	Ill.	N.Y.
Wis.	Pa.		Tex.	Iowa	R.I.
	Tenn.		Utah	Me.	
	Va.			Miss.	
	Vt.			N.C.	
	Wash.			S.C.	
				W. Va.	

Source: *American Medical Directory*, 6th ed. (1918), pp. 175–1685, passim, with occasional use made of the 5th ed. (1916).

APPENDIX V. "A GENERAL PLAN FOR A SCHEDULE OF MEDICAL FEES" by J. N. McCormack (Abstract)

Purposes of a Schedule

1. TO MEET THE HAZARDS OF INFLATION. "With the cost of living almost

doubled and the cost of equipment for modern practice quadrupled, the income of medical men, except surgeons and specialists, has remained almost stationary."

2. TO RAISE THE EARNING POWER OF INFERIOR PHYSICIANS. "What is first and most needed in dealing with this class, for their own good as well as of the people, is to raise their earning capacity to make them better practitioners and better men, by means of consistent, persistent postgraduate study, and by the influence and example of the higher grade members in every county society and in such intercourse as comes in daily practice, and then in leading them to the adoption of systematic business methods and aiding them in other ways in securing better compensation."

3. TO PROMOTE PUBLIC WELFARE. "Properly interpreted, poverty in the profession, and the lack of equipment and practical incompetency inseparable from it, is just as important to the public as to us, and the subject should be boldly discussed in public meetings and in the periodical and daily press until the real positive danger to the people is a matter of common knowledge."

4. TO ALLOW FOR CHARITY WORK. "To an extent not dreamed of by the laity, or even by many in the higher ranks of the profession, a large per cent, of the physicians in this country, in cities and towns as well as in the rural districts, on account of poverty and the pressing needs of their own families, are daily forced to take what is almost blood money from a class of widows, teachers and working women, in their times of affliction, whose incomes are so scanty when well, that it would and should be an honor and a pleasure to make them the special wards and beneficiaries of a properly supported profession."

"Schedule of Medical Fees for _____ County

1. Day visit in town	$ 2.00
2. Night visit in town	3.00
3. Day visit in country, first mile, $2.00; each after mile, one way	1.00
4. Night visit in country, first mile, $3.00; each after mile, one way	1.50
5. Ordinary office examination and advice	1.00
6. Complete examination and advice	5.00
7. Advice or prescription by telephone	1.00
8. Obstetric case, uncomplicated, not over 6 hours	15.00
9. Life insurance examinations	5.00
10. Consultation, double ordinary visit	
11. Surgical and other special fees as may be arranged	

Explanatory Note (Extracts)

"This schedule of fees is purely advisory. It is arranged and published for the information and guidance equally of the profession and people. It is intended to suggest the fees for ordinary services by competent physicians, for these fully able to pay their bills. It in no way applies to practice for the deserving poor, of which all agree to do their full part. It may be that physicians who are less competent will feel that they should charge less for their services. This is recognized as just, and to do so will in no way affect either their society membership or professional standing."

Source: *JAMA* 51 (28 Nov. 1908): 1882–83.

APPENDIX VI. "ARTICLES OF AGREEMENT" Carlisle County (Kentucky) Medical Society, December 3, 1907

Agreement made between the Carlisle County Medical Society and the members thereof, as follows:

We, the undersigned members of the Carlisle County Medical Society, of Carlisle County, Kentucky, hereby agree and bind ourselves, subject to the penalties named herein:

First: Each member shall submit to the Secretary of this society the names of persons who have persistently refused or neglected to settle their accounts for medical services rendered within a reasonable period, and such other names from time to time as each member may think to their interest.

Second: The names submitted as per section first shall be arranged alphabetically, to be known as the "Information List," and each member of this society shall be assigned a number by which he shall be known in the list.

Third: Every member of this society shall be furnished a copy of the "Information List." All names reported by the secretary shall be added or removed as reported.

Fourth: It shall be the duty of each member of this society to inform any person whose name appears in the "Information List" apply[ing] to them for medical services, that they owe an account to the physician or physicians reporting their names. Exceptions to this rule may be made as follows: In case of emergency the physician applied to may render immediate medical aid to the extent of one visit to such person, providing the physician rendering the service demands and receives cash payment for the service; but shall refuse further services except for cash or a written voucher signed by some legally responsible person for the payment of same.

Fifth: The person so reported may make application to the physician or physicians reporting his name, pay the amount due, or make satisfactory arrangements for the payment thereof. Then it shall be the duty of the physician reporting said person to issue a certificate on the form prescribed by this society, certifying that he had paid the account or made other satisfactory arrangements for the payment of the same. In this event, it shall be the privilege of any physician to whom said person shall apply and present said certificate, to render medical services.

Sixth: In the event of a person receiving a certificate of satisfactory arrangements for settlement of his account failing to comply with his agreement made in order to receive said certificate, the name shall again be placed on the "Information List," and each and every member of the society shall refuse absolutely to render further medical services until the terms of said agreement have been complied with or a new certificate issued.

Seventh: The following form of certificate shall be used for the purpose set forth in section sixth:

This certifies that Mr. _____ has this day agreed to settle his account of $_____ by making payment on the _____ day of each and every _____ until said account is settled in full. Date _____ 19_____

Signed

_____ M.D.

Eighth: It shall be the duty of each and every member of this society to render statements to his patrons quarterly on the first day of January, April, July and October of each year. Privilege is hereby granted to render monthly statements.

Ninth: It shall be compulsory upon each and every member of this society to comply with the conditions of this agreement, also to abide by the minimum fees as set forth in the fee bill adopted, also the code of ethics; and upon trial and conviction before the Censors of the Carlisle County Medical Society pay a fine of from $5 to $10; or expulsion from the society shall be imposed upon any member who wilfully or negligently refuses to comply with the conditions herein set forth.

(Signed)
MEMBERS

Note: This society adopted the agreement and a revised fee schedule both signed by fourteen physicians.
Source: *Ky. Med. Jour.* 6 (Feb. 1908): 103–4.

APPENDIX VII. OBJECTIONS TO COMPULSORY HEALTH INSUR-
ANCE DRAFTED BY THE COMMITTEE ON SOCIAL OR HEALTH
INSURANCE OF THE CHICAGO MEDICAL SOCIETY AND EN-
DORSED BY THE COMMITTEE ON HEALTH INSURANCE OF
THE ILLINOIS MEDICAL SOCIETY
(An Abstract)

1. "Organized labor, the employer of labor, the taxpayer and the physician . . . are unequivocally opposed to it."

2. In this bill of the American Association for Labor Legislation the social reformer calls only for sickness insurance "while with equal arguments and authority he attempts to prove the necessity of invalidity insurance, old-age insurance and death insurance by state provision."

3. "No new health insurance legislation should be enacted before we rectify the unfairness of the present [workmen's] compensation law."

4. Present system of treating the poor by the "most efficient medical men" is far superior to medical service in areas providing health insurance.

5. Poverty is the cause of sickness and sickness is not the cause of poverty.

6. Health insurance would increase poverty "by shifting the burden of paying a living wage and giving steady employment from the place where it belongs."

7. Prohibition, soon to become effective in Illinois, will largely eliminate the need for health insurance, if one exists, by diverting sufficient income toward payment of medical bills.

8. Health insurance has been unsatisfactory in Germany and England and the "weight of learned opinion" opposes it in France.

9. It will not solve the abuse of medical charity. "The physician's charity list is made up of those who are not provided for in this bill."

10. It will enlarge medical charity adding 240,000 "who, through physical unfitness or old age, will be driven to involuntary idleness through the operation of this bill."

11. It is inadequate since it provides medical service only for the "unusually healthy."

12. "Selection of employees would cease to be based upon efficiency and value to the employer . . . but upon the state of health and presumptive continuance of this good health." The bill would encourage employers to establish "physical standards as yet undreamed of," and would "create a very large number of cast-offs, who virtually become non-wage-earning derelicts, but for whose support no provision is made in the proposed law." Illinois would confront the problem of providing "employment or a living for the 8 per cent or 192,000 physically defective wage-earner discards. After those were provided for, it could do the same for the 2 per cent, or 48,000, perfectly good wage-earners 55 years of age or over who would be rejected by the carrier associations."

13. It would impose a burden on the casual worker who would remain unprotected because of poverty or because of "general incompetence previous illness or any other disabling condition."

14. It would place a premium on inferior medical care offering its greatest rewards to the least efficient physicians.

15. It would encourage superfluous service. "As long as there is a quantitative relationship between services and compensation, superfluous services are inevitable."

16. It would encourage secret conniving between panel physicians and panel specialists. "The general practitioner will be at the mercy of the medical officer or cliques of doctors organized into hospitals."

17. "Certain physicians will underbid the panel physicians, and with the insurance companies and funds to back them, will compel the commission by law to accept their bids."

18. "It will convert the practice of medicine into a vast kind of lodge practice (with all of its evils)."

19. It threatens the ethics of the profession. "The physician who will lengthen the period of disability for the patient will be the most popular and financially successful; the physician of conscience and ability, refusing to conform to the professional and moral status of the unscrupulous, will be forced to penury or forced out of the profession of medicine."

20. It would standardize medical practice "to an intolerable degree of inferiority."

21. It will "stop scientific progress in medical research . . . by destroying the incentive for research and individual excellence."

22. It could not function successfully with a dissatisfied medical profession.

23. It would create much malingering.

24. It would destroy the confidential relationship between the physician and the patient.

25. It would not improve public health.

26. It would divide the public into classes.

27. It would inflict moral injury on the beneficiaries. "It lessens the public ideals of truthfulness and honesty, destroys the spirit of personal independence and increases the moral trend toward pauperism."

28. "We believe in health insurance for the wage-earner, but we believe that he should pay for it, and that it should not be 40 per cent purchase and 60 per cent charity.

29. "It is another scheme to exploit the profession by the community."

30. The layman is as much entitled to state-provided legal service as to medical service. If the state is to "coddle" some wage-earners why should it not also "establish farms to furnish produce, mines to furnish coal, mills and factories to furnish all wearing apparel at cost [?]"

31. It will not effect much of an economic saving by redeeming the "waste of time-value" stressed by insurance proponents.

32. It will inflict enormous operational costs on the state.

33. It will create a powerful bureaucracy "that would have some degree of contact or authority over all of the workers of the state."

34. It will require some 1,000 carrier associations, many of which "would be politically organized, equipped and controlled."

35. It does not provide for comprehensive coverage, security, or plan solvency, and provides no protection against many operational abuses.

36. It provides for "paternalistic government of the rankest kind," and is opposed to the "spirit of American institutions."

37. In requiring citizens to enter the system against their will and assume the burden of premiums it is "un-American."

38. "The adoption of compulsory health insurance would mark the beginning of a socialistic state, under which all rights of the individual are subordinated."

Note: These objections have been numbered and consolidated for convenience.
Source: *Ill. Med. Jour.* 31 (March 1917); 188–94.

BIBLIOGRAPHICAL ESSAY

The Progressive Era marks the period when most of the state medical associations converted their annual volumes of transactions into journals, established monthly journals, or adopted a private publication as their official organ. The Pennsylvania society led the way in 1896, adopting a private journal as its official publication. The Illinois society followed with its journal in 1898, and in 1900 the Kansas Medical Society and the New York State Medical Association established journals. By November 1905 ten other state associations and one territorial society had established their own organs. These included societies in Arkansas, Kentucky, Michigan, Missouri, New Jersey, Ohio, Texas, California, Colorado, South Carolina, and the Territory of New Mexico. By June 1909 the societies in Indiana, Maryland, Oklahoma, Tennessee, and West Virginia had established journals, raising the total with official organs to twenty-one. At the end of 1917, twenty-seven state societies had such journals, which actually served societies in thirty-five states.

This volume rests in a large measure on exhaustive or substantial research in the transactions, journals and other published records of the societies in every geographical division of the nation. In New England and the Middle Atlantic States the societies included in this research are Massachusetts, New York, and Pennsylvania; in the South Atlantic States, the societies in Maryland and South Carolina. Societies in the East North Central States include those in Illinois, Michigan, and Wisconsin; in the East South Central, Alabama, Kentucky, and Tennessee. In the West North Central, the list includes societies in Missouri and Kansas; in the West South Central, Louisiana and Texas. Among the Pacific States the California society is included; its journal also served as the official organ of the Nevada society toward the close of the Progressive Era. The societies of Washington, Oregon, and Utah are represented in this research through their official organ, *Northwest Medicine*. The published records of many other local, state, and regional societies have been examined, as well as the American Medical Association's *Journal* and several other of its publications.

The literature of irregular medical and healing groups is substantial. Treatment of the homeopathic movement rests largely on the *Transactions of the American Institute of Homeopathy,* the *Journal of the American Institute of Homeopathy,* and the *Hahnemannian Monthly,* although a number of other homeopathic publications were examined and several are cited. The *Eclectic Medical Journal* and the *National Eclectic Medical Association Quarterly* provided most of the information for the treatment of the eclectic system, but several other publications reflecting eclectic views were examined. The *Journal of the American Osteopathic Association* and the *Journal of Osteopathy* constituted principal sources for information on the osteopathic movement. For the chiropractic movement reliance has been placed largely on published works of chiropractors and their critics, while standard monographs and periodical literature have been used for dealing with other healing groups.

Several private collections were important for this study. On medical education I used the Flexner Papers, Manuscripts Division of the Library of Congress; William H. Welch Papers at the Johns Hopkins Institute of the History of Medicine; the George Blumer Papers and the Harvey Cushing Materials in the Yale Medical Historical Library; and at the Rockefeller Archive Center, Hillcrest, Pocantico Hills, North Tarrytown, New York, research in the Frederick T. Gates Papers, the Edwin Embree Papers, and some of the files of the General Education Board was rewarding. For irregular groups, the J. U. Lloyd Letter Collection, Cincinnati Historical Library, and the limited materials examined in the A. T. Still File, Library of the Kirksville College of Osteopathy and Surgery, were of some help. On the social insurance issue the John B. Andrews Papers and the Max M. Rubinow Papers in the Library of the New York State School of Industrial and Labor Relations, Cornell University, were invaluable.

ABBREVIATIONS

American Academy of Medicine	Amer. Acad. Med.
American Homeopathist	Amer. Homeop.
American Labor Legislation Review	Amer. Labor Leg. Rev.
American Medical Association Bulletin	AMA Bulletin
American Medical Compend.	Amer. Med. Comp.
American Medicine	Amer. Med.
American Medical Directory	Amer. Med. Dir.
American Medical Monthly	Amer. Med. Monthly
Boston Medical and Surgical Journal	Boston Med. Surg. Jour.
British Medical Journal	British Med. Jour.
Bulletin of the American Academy of Medicine	Bull. Amer. Acad. Med.
Bulletin of the History of Medicine	Bull. Hist. Med.
California Eclectic Medical Journal	Calif. Eclectic Med. Jour.
California State Journal of Medicine	Calif. St. Jour. Med.
Colorado Medical Journal	Colo. Med. Jour.
Colorado Medical Journal and Western Medical and Surgical Gazette	Colo. Med. Jour. and Western Gaz.
Delaware State Medical Journal	Del. St. Med. Jour.
Eclectic Medical Gleaner	Eclectic Med. Gleaner
Eclectic Medical Journal	Eclectic Med. Jour.
Eclectic Medical News	Eclectic Med. News
Eclectic Review	Eclectic Rev.
Hahnemannian Monthly	Hahne. Monthly
Homeopathic Recorder	Homeop. Recorder
Illinois Medical Journal	Ill. Med. Jour.
Indiana Medical Journal	Ind. Med. Jour.
Journal of the American Institute of Homeopathy	Jour. AIH
Journal of the American Medical Association	JAMA
Journal of the American Osteopathic Association	Jour. Amer. Osteop. Assn.
Journal of the History of Medicine and Allied Sciences	Jour. Hist. Med.
Journal of the Kansas Medical Society	Jour. Kans. Med. Soc.
Journal of the Kansas Medical Society in Which Is Incorporated the Wichita Medical Journal	Jour. Kans. Med. Soc. and Wichita Med. Jour.
Journal of the Medical Society of the State of New Jersey	Jour. Med. Soc. St. N.J.

Journal of the Michigan State Medical Society	Jour. Mich. St. Med. Soc.
Journal of the Missouri State Medical Association	Jour. Mo. St. Med. Assn.
Journal of the Oklahoma Medical Association	Jour. Okla. Med. Assn.
Journal of Osteopathy	Jour. Osteop.
Journal of the South Carolina Medical Association	Jour. S.C. Med. Assn.
Journal of the State Medical Society of the State of New Jersey	Jour. St. Med. Soc. St. N.J.
Kentucky Medical Journal	Ky. Med. Jour.
Los Angeles Journal of Eclectic Medicine	L.A. Jour. Eclectic Med.
Long Island Medical Journal	Long Island Med. Jour.
Maryland Medical Journal	Md. Med. Jour.
Medical Communications of the Massachusetts Medical Society	Med. Com. Mass. Med. Soc.
Medical Century	Med. Century
Medical and Surgical Gazette	Med. Surg. Gaz.
Medical Record	Med. Record
Medical World	Med. World
National Chiropractic	Nat. Chirop.
National Eclectic Medical Association Quarterly	Nat. Eclectic Med. Assn. Quar.
New England Medical Gazette	N.E. Med. Gaz.
New Orleans Medical and Surgical Journal	New Orleans Med. Surg. Jour.
New York Medical Journal	N.Y. Med. Jour.
New York State Journal of Medicine	N.Y. St. Jour. Med.
Northwest Medicine	Northwest Med.
Occidental Medical Times	Occid. Med. Times
Ohio State Medical Journal	Ohio St. Med. Jour.
Oklahoma State Medical Association Journal	Okla. St. Med. Assn. Jour.
Pennsylvania Medical Journal	Pa. Med. Jour.
Southern Medical Journal	Southern Med. Jour.
St. Paul Medical Journal	St. Paul Med. Jour.
Texas State Journal of Medicine	Texas St. Jour. Med.
Wisconsin Medical Journal	Wis. Med. Jour.

NOTES

CHAPTER ONE

1. *New York Times*, 31 Dec. 1899, p. 8, Editorial, p. 20. This volume follows the plan of the federal census in concluding a decade with next to the last decennial year although, of course, 1 January 1901 actually marked the first day of the twentieth century. But for public confusion over whether the new century began on 1 January 1900 or 1 January 1901, see Paul F. Boller, Jr., *American Thought in Transition: The Impact of Evolutionary Naturalism, 1865–1900* (Chicago: Rand McNally & Co., 1969), pp. 227–29; Walter Lord, *The Good Years: from 1900 to the First World War* (New York: Harper & Brothers, 1960), p. 1, and *Abilene* [Texas] *Reporter News*, morning edition (1 Jan. 1976), p. 6–A. The editorial in the *Times* recognized 1900 as the last year of the century, but ignored the Boer and Philippine conflicts, although factual coverage of the Boer War appears on the first page and a rather curious note on "The Religion of the Boers" on the editorial page.

2. C. C. Regier, *The Era of the Muckrakers* (Chapel Hill: University of North Carolina Press, 1932), pp. 27–31, 51.

3. Ibid., p. 22. For Roosevelt's use of the term "muckraker" and his explanation see ibid., pp. 1–2.

4. Ibid., pp. 55, 47, 135–36, 181–82; James G. Burrow, *AMA: Voice of American Medicine* (Baltimore: The Johns Hopkins Press, 1963), pp. 67–83. For an excellent treatment of the general climate producing federal food and drug legislation see James Harvey Young, *The Toadstool Millionaires: A Social History of Patent Medicine in America before Federal Regulation* (Princeton: Princeton University Press, 1962), and for division among railroads and with shippers on regulatory measures see Robert H. Weibe, *Businessmen and Reform* (Cambridge: Harvard University Press, 1962), pp. 14–15, 51–56.

5. Regier, *Era of Muckrakers*, pp. 126–31, 111–14; Harold U. Faulkner, *The Decline of Laissez Faire, 1897–1917*, The Economic History of the United States, vol. 7, ed. Henry David et al. (New York: Harper & Row, 1951), pp. 256–61, 266–70; Josephine Goldmark, *Impatient Crusader* (Urbana: University of Illinois Press, 1953), pp. 78–92, 132–72, passim.

6. Stubbs's address, *Transactions of the State Medical Association of Texas*, 33d ann. sess. (Galveston, 1901), p. 9; quotation, H. A. West, "Medical and Sociological Aspects of the Galveston Storm," ibid., p. 118; Walter B. Stevens, "The Story of the Galveston Disaster," *Munsey's Magazine* 24 (Dec. 1900): 347. West was not only a prominent Texas physician but had been elected vice president of the American Medical Association in 1898. For further information about his career see *JAMA* 42

(16 Jan. 1904): 184, and George Plunket Red (Mrs. S. C. Red), *The Medical Man in Texas* (Houston: Standard Printing and Lithographing Co., 1930), pp. 224–25.

7. West, "Medical and Sociological Aspects," p. 118; Alvah H. Doty, "The Mosquito: Its Relation to Disease and Its Extermination," *N.Y. St. Jour. Med.* 8 (May 1908): 225; Rudolph Matas, "A Communication," *New Orleans Med. Surg. Jour.* 64 (May 1914): 827; H. A. West, "Further Observations on the Medical Aspects of the Galveston Storm," *Trans. St. Med. Assn. Texas,* 1901, p. 135.

8. "The Report of the Government Commission on the Existence of Plague in San Francisco," *Occid. Med. Times* 15 (April 1901): 101–17; James H. Parkinson, Resolution, ibid., p. 301; Editorial, ibid. 15 (May 1901): 171; Editorial, *Calif. St. Jour. Med.* 5 (Dec. 1907): 301; Editorial, ibid. 6 (Feb. 1908): 38; *Transactions of the Medical Society of the State of California,* 31st. ann. sess., 30 (Sacramento, 1901): 60–61, 86–87, 367.

9. Charles F. MacDonald, "The Trial, Execution, Autopsy, and Mental Status of Leon F. Czolgosz, Alias Fred Nieman, the Assassin of President McKinley," *N.Y. Med. Jour.* 75 (4 Jan. 1902): 12, quotation, p. 13.

10. "The Post-Mortem Examination of Leon F. Czolgosz," *N.Y. Med. Jour.* 75 (4 Jan. 1902): 23.

11. The Rockefeller Foundation, International Health Board, *Bibliography of Hookworm Disease, Publication No. 11* (New York, 1922), p. xix; Wm. W. Dinsmore, "Hookworm Disease a National Problem," *Transactions of the Medical Association of the State of Alabama* (State Board of Health) (Mobile, 1913), p. 466.

12. Bernard Wolff, "Are Jews Immune to Pellagra?" *Southern Med. Jour.* 5 (March 1912): 119. For accounts of the origin and spread of this disease see J. M. King, "Pellagra, with a Report of Cases," ibid. 1 (Nov. 1908): 292–93, and the comprehensive treatment in Elizabeth W. Etheridge, *The Butterfly Caste: A Social History of Pellagra in the South* (Westport, Conn.: Greenwood Pub. Co., 1972), esp. pp. 3–39.

13. George W. Webster, "Pellagra, with Special Reference to Etiology and Diagnosis," *Ill. Med. Jour.* 18 (Aug. 1910): 140; "Attempts to Produce Experimental Pellagra," *Scientific American* 104 (2 Dec. 1911): 490; *New Orleans Med. Surg. Jour.* 63 (Nov. 1910): 377; C. C. Bass, Remarks, ibid. 65 (Nov. 1912): 383, 385; Chilton Thorington, "Some Suggestions on the Etiology of Pellagra," ibid. 64 (Sept. 1911): 183; "On the Track of a Pellagra Cure," *Literary Digest* 50 (20 March 1915): 604; Benjamin Brooks, "Mountains—The Cause of Pellagra," *Illustrated World* 26 (1 Jan. 1916): 644; "Corn and Pellagra," *American Review of Reviews* 41 (March 1910): 351; Editorial, *Southern Med. Jour.* 2 (Jan. 1909): 461; "Food and Pellagra," *Survey* 36 (27 May 1916): 223; *Scientific American Supplement* 81 (1 Jan. 1916): 11; *New Orleans Med. Surg. Jour.* 67 (Dec. 1914): 576.

14. Henry P. de Forest, "Prostitution," *N.Y. St. Jour. Med.* 8 (Oct. 1908): 529; Editorial, *Ind. Med. Jour.* 21 (March 1903): 377–78; A. W. Brayton and Charles E. Ferguson, Remarks, ibid. 21 (May 1903): 457; Seneca Egbert, "Typhoid Fever in Pennsylvania," *Pa. Med. Jour.* 9 (Feb. 1906): 324. Many other states reported smallpox cases in the early twentieth century, but the Indiana epidemic seems to have been the most severe. See also Editorial, *Ill. Med. Jour.* 3 (April 1902): 531.

15. Herman Oechsner, Remarks, *New Orleans Med. Surg. Jour.* 67 (July 1914): 49; Robert W. Lovett, "The Occurrence of Infantile Paralysis in Massachusetts in 1907," *Med. Com. Mass. Med. Soc.* 21, no. 3 (Boston, 1910): 784; Edward Francis, "History of Tularaemia," The Johns Hopkins University School of Hygiene and Public Health, *De Lamar Lectures, 1926–1927* (Baltimore: Williams and Wilkins Co., 1928), pp. 94, 102. See also William L. Jellison, "Tularemia: Dr.

Edward Francis and His First 23 Isolates," *Bull. Hist. Med.* 46 (Sept.–Oct. 1972): 447, 478.

16. Monroe Lerner and Odin W. Anderson, *Health Progress in the United States, 1900–1950* (Chicago: University of Chicago Press, 1963), pp. 15–16.

17. *JAMA* 40 (9 May 1903): 1273. For another admission of the limitations of curative medicine see Frederick C. Shattuck, "The Value of Drugs in Therapeutics," *Boston Med. Surg. Jour.* 154 (22 March 1906): 333, and for a recommendation of bloodletting in some cases of pneumonia as late as 1914 see Hugh Boyd, "Blood-Letting in Pneumonia," *Transactions of the Medical Association of the State of Alabama* (Montgomery, 1914), p. 316.

18. Frederic P. Gorham, "The History of Bacteriology and Its Contribution to Public Health Work," in Mazyck P. Ravenel, ed., *A Half Century of Public Health* (New York: American Public Health Association, 1921), pp. 71–72; J. H. Mason Knox, "The Growth of Our Knowledge of Infectious Diseases," *Md. Med. Jour.* 51 (June 1908): 216–19; S. B. Wolbach, "The Filterable Viruses," *Med. Com. Mass. Med. Soc.* 23 (Boston, 1912): 327.

19. Richard Harrison Shryock, *The Development of Modern Medicine* (New York: Alfred A. Knopf, 1947), pp. 289, 290, 301–2; Edwin H. Ackerknecht, *A Short History of Medicine* (New York: Ronald Press Co., 1955), pp. 168, 221; *Texas St. Jour. Med.* 9 (Jan. 1914): 284.

20. Ackerknecht, *History of Medicine*, p. 221; C. D. Haagensen and Wyndham W. B. Lloyd, *A Hundred Years of Medicine* (New York: Sheridan House, 1943), pp. 70–73, 352–55, 144, 265, 306–7, 311, 316, 323–25, 207; Shryock, *Modern Medicine*, p. 369; *British Med. Jour.* (19 Nov. 1910): 1606–7. Other medical achievements of the Progressive period are well summarized in David L. Cohen, *Medicine and Health in New Jersey: A History* (Princeton: D. Van Nostrand Co.), pp. 113–15.

21. Charles Singer and E. Ashworth Underwood, *A Short History of Medicine* (New York: Oxford University Press, 1962), pp. 612, 637; Haagesen and Lloyd, *Hundred Years of Medicine*, p. 262; Ackerknecht, *History of Medicine*, p. 213.

22. *JAMA* 35 (29 Sept. 1900): 834–35; Editorial, *N.Y. Med. Jour.* 72 (29 Sept. 1900): 550–51, see also pp. 555–56; Ackerknecht, *History of Medicine*, p. 207; Haagensen and Lloyd, *Hundred Years of Medicine*, pp. 309, 314; *Md. Med. Jour.* 18 (Oct. 1900): 530; *Ind. Med. Jour.* 19 (Oct. 1900): 157–58.

23. Editorial, *Ill. Med. Jour.* 3 (April 1902): 532; *JAMA* 42 (25 June 1904): 1691–92; *N.Y. Med. Jour.* 87 (11 Jan. 1908): 75. For an evaluation of Fenger's work see George Rosen, "Christian Fenger: Medical Immigrant," *Bull. Hist. Med.* 48 (Spring 1974): 129–45.

24. Ackernecht, *History of Medicine*, p. 209; Loyal Davis, *J. B. Murphy: Stormy Petrel of Surgery* (New York: G. P. Putnam's Sons, 1938), pp. 238–42, 246–47; Helen B. Clapseattle, *The Doctors Mayo* (Minneapolis: University of Minnesota Press, 1941), p. 533; Arthur E. Hertzler, *The Horse and Buggy Doctor* (New York: Harper & Brothers, 1938), pp. 212–13, 265, 277.

25. Haagensen and Lloyd, *Hundred Years of Medicine*, pp. 172–73, 324–25.

26. Joseph Rilus Eastman, Remarks, *Ind. Med. Jour.* 21 (June 1903): 515; Editorial, *Md. Med. Jour.* 46 (Jan. 1903): 41–42; Editorial, *Colo. Med. Jour.* 2 (15 Nov. 1906): 237.

27. Charles A. L. Reed, "Rudolph Virchow: An Appreciation," *Transactions of the Medical Society of the State of New York*, 97th ann. sess. (Albany, 1903), pp. 59–76; *Ind. Med. Jour.* 21 (Oct. 1902), 178; *N.Y. Med. Jour.* 87 (18 April 1908): 748–49; Davis, *J. B. Murphy*, pp. 240–41. For a high tribute to Murphy upon his death and for his stature in world medicine see Editorial, *Md. Med. Jour.* 59 (Sept.

1916), 231. The flow of Americans to European medical schools after 1870 and the visitations of prominent European physicians to the United States early in the twentieth century is described in Thomas Neville Bonner, *American Doctors and German Universities: A Chapter in International Intellectual Relations, 1870–1910* (Lincoln: University of Nebraska Press, 1963), esp. pp. 23, 69, 73, 139–56.

28. James Howard Means, *The Association of American Physicians* (New York: McGraw-Hill, 1961), p. 84; F. Emerson Andrews, *Philanthropic Foundations* (New York: Russell Sage Foundation, 1956), p. 40; Carnegie Institution of Washington, *Yearbook*, No. 1, 1902 (Washington: Published by the Institution, 1903), pp. vii, viii; Editorial, *Ill. Med. Jour.* 5 (Aug. 1903): 172. For a list of the foundations established for medical research see "Report of the Committee on Medical Research," *Proceedings of the Association of American Medical Colleges, Twenty-Seventh Annual Meeting* (Chicago, 1917), p. 22.

29. *Md. Med. Jour.* 45 (April 1902): 185; Nelson D. Brayton, Remarks, *Ind. Med. Jour.* 20 (April 1902): 371; *Amer. Med.*, n.s. 2 (Aug. 1907): 488.

30. Editorial, *New Orleans Med. Surg. Jour.* 66 (Jan. 1914): 560; Editorial, ibid. 67 (July 1914): 69; Haagensen and Lloyd, *Hundred Years of Medicine*, p. 383.

CHAPTER TWO

1. Arthur E. Hertzler, *The Horse and Buggy Doctor* (New York: Harper & Brothers, 1938), pp. 117–18.

2. Richard Hofstadter, *The Age of Reform* (New York: Alfred A. Knopf, 1955), pp. 148–64.

3. Editorial, *St. Paul Med. Jour.* 12 (July 1910): 341. Another journal observed that some other groups shared the financial disadvantages of most physicians, stating that "the hardships of the medical profession are by no means peculiar. They are shared to a greater or less degree by other professions and by small capitalists and business men generally." This quotation from *Medical Times* appears in *Amer. Med. Compend.* 26 (Feb. 1910): 45. For a convincing presentation of the case that the workers' real wages had declined between 1900 and 1914 see Isaac M. Rubinow, "The Recent Trend of Real Wages," reprint from the *American Economic Review* 4 (Dec. 1914): 817. For ample protestations of the profession's economic distress see Editorial, *Texas St. Jour. Med.* 1 (Nov. 1905): 157–58; T. M. Johnson, "The Business Side of the Practice of Medicine," *Ohio St. Med. Jour.* 1 (15 June 1906): 582; G. R. Waite, Remarks, *Jour. Kans. Med. Soc.* 7 (1 Nov. 1907), 1136; *Pa. Med. Jour.* 11 (Feb. 1908): 382, quoting J. F. Blanchard in *Vermont Medical Monthly* (15 Nov. 1907); James E. Murray, "Business and Ethics in Their Relation to the Practice of Medicine," address summarized by R. H. Greebe, *Ohio St. Med. Jour.* 5 (15 Jan. 1909): 38; H. H. McCarthy, "Some of the Evils of Medical Practice," *Northwest Med.*, n.s. 2 (March 1910) 89; Theodore W. Schaeffer and Albert M. Wilson, "Expert Medical Evidence at One Dollar Per Day," *New Orleans Med. Surg. Jour.* 62 (June 1910): 992; Editorial, *Texas St. Jour. Med.* 12 (Jan. 1917): 379–80.

4. Borden S. Veeder, "Standards for Determining the Suitability of Patients for Admission to a Free Dispensary," *JAMA* 67 (8 July 1916): 87; *Colo. Med. Jour. and Western Gaz.* 8 (Aug. 1902): 150, citing an editorial from *Medical World*.

5. Edgar Allen Forbes, "Is the Doctor a Shylock?" *World's Work* 14 (May 1907): 8892–96; "Secretary's Report," *Texas St. Jour. Med.* 3 (June 1907): 65. The last citation incorrectly gives 55 instead of 52 percent as barely making a living. For the extent of inflation and for an estimate of $650 to $800 as being the minimum living cost for the urban family of a workingman about 1910 see Harold U. Faulkner, *The Decline of Laissez Faire, 1897–1917*, The Economic History of the United

States, vol. 7, ed. Henry David et. al. (New York: Rinehart & Co. 1951), pp. 252, 255.

6. George H. Simmons, "Medical Education and Preliminary Requirements," *JAMA* 42 (7 May 1904): 1205. For examples of complaints over a surplus of physicians see Frank Billings, "Medical Education in the United States," *JAMA* 40 (9 May 1903): 1272; J. N. McCormack, "The Status of Organization in Missouri," *Jour. Mo. St. Med. Assn.* 2 (Jan. 1905): 31; "Report of the Council on Medical Education," *ibid.* 7 (July 1910): 30; H. S. Delamere to editor, *Calif. St. Jour. Med.* 2 (Jan. 1904): 30; ibid. 6 (Aug. 1908): 270; T. N. Rafferty, "The Present Status of the General Practitioner," *Ill. Med. Jour.* 7 (Jan. 1905): 50; V. Berry, "President's Address," *Joint Session of the Oklahoma State Medical Association with the Indian Territorial Medical Association* (Oklahoma City, 1906), p. 33. For an expression of doubt about the surplus quite at variance with the citations above see Editorial, *Jour. Mo. St. Med. Assn.* 3 (Sept. 1904): 142. For views of irregular healing sects see chapter 5.

7. For a discussion of the laxity of control over medical education see chapter 3, and for a brief account of state licensing laws in the late nineteenth century although based on sources not wholly accurate see Jeffrey Lionel Berlant, *Profession and Monopoly* (Berkeley: University of California Press, 1975), pp. 234–35.

8. J. N. McCormack, "The Organization of the Medical Profession," *Northwest Med.* 3 (Oct. 1905): 293.

9. [Arthur T. McCormack], "Some Personal Sketches," *Ky. Med. Jour.* 21 (Jan. 1923): 20–22.

10. Ibid., pp. 22–23.

11. J. N. McCormack, "The Organization of the Minnesota State Medical Association," *Transactions of the Minnesota State Medical Association*, 35th ann. sess. (Minneapolis, 1903), p. 42; quotation, James N. Baker, "President's Message," *Transactions of the Medical Association of the State of Alabama* (State Board of Health) (Montgomery, 1916), p. 1601.

12. W. H. Sanders, "The History, Philosophy and Fruits of Medical Organization in Alabama," *Transactions of the Medical Association of the State of Alabama* (Montgomery, 1914), pp. 521, 526–35, 660–61; McCormack, "Organization of the Medical Profession," p. 295. For societies granted the licensing power in the late eighteenth and early nineteenth centuries see Joseph F. Kett, *The Formation of the American Medical Profession* (New Haven: Yale University Press, 1968), pp. 181–84.

13. Charles A. L. Reed, "President's Address," *JAMA* 36 (8 June 1901): 1604; *Transactions of the Medical Association of the State of Alabama* (Montgomery, 1902), pp. 17, 20.

14. J. N. McCormack, "Organization and Its Advantages to the Individual Doctor," *Texas St. Jour. Med.* 1 (Jan. 1906): 225. This address was imperfectly reproduced from the editor's notes but McCormack frequently used this or similar phraseology.

15. J. N. McCormack, "Things about Doctors Which Doctors and Other People Ought to Know," *Jour. Mich. St. Med. Soc.* 6 (Jan. 1907): 32.

16. Editorial, *Ky. Med. Jour.* 14 (1 June 1916): 292.

17. McCormack, "Organization and Its Advantages," p. 225.

18. Ibid.

19. Ibid., pp. 226–27; McCormack, "Organization of the Minnesota State Medical Association," p. 52.

20. J. N. McCormack, "The Great Work Being Done in Texas," *JAMA* 46 (April 1906): 1134; McCormack, "Organization and Its Advantages," p. 225.

21. J. N. McCormack, "About the Discord Still Existing in Some County Societies," *Ky. Med. Jour.* 14 (1 June 1916): 292; McCormack, "Things about Doctors," p. 36.

22. McCormack, "Organization and Its Advantages," p. 229.

23. James G. Burrow, *AMA: Voice of American Medicine* (Baltimore: The Johns Hopkins Press, 1963), p. 39. For an example of situations McCormack encountered that combined friendliness and friction, see J. N. McCormack, "Oregon Practically an Unorganized State," *JAMA* 45 (9 Dec. 1905): 1818–19.

24. McCormack, "Organization and Its Advantages," p. 228.

25. McCormack, "Things about Doctors," pp. 33, 36–37; McCormack, "Organization and Its Advantages," p. 228; J. N. McCormack, "A General Plan for a Schedule of Medical Fees," *JAMA* 51 (28 Nov. 1908): 1882–83. For a citation of a state journal to this plan see *Ill. Med. Jour.* 15 (Feb. 1909): 205–9.

26. McCormack, "Organization and Its Advantages," p. 227; *Trans. Minn. St. Med. Assn.*, 1903, p. 15; *Pa. Med. Jour.* 12 (May 1909): 649–54; I. V. Chase, "Secretary's Report," *Texas St. Jour. Med.* 3 (June 1907): 62; E. T. Shelby to editor, *Jour. Kans. Med. Soc.* 5 (1 April 1905): 165; "Report of the Proceedings of the Council," *Transactions of the Indiana State Medical Association*, 56th ann. sess. (Indianapolis, 1905), p. 475; *Texas St. Jour. Med.* 2 (May 1906): 15; D. C. Moriarta, Report, *N. Y. St. Jour. Med.* 8 (Feb. 1908): 93; M. A. Clark, "President's Address," *Transactions of the Medical Association of Georgia*, 60th ann. sess. (Atlanta, 1909), p. 29; *Jour. Mo. St. Med. Assn.* 8 (July 1911): 29.

27. Wilfred Haughey, "Post-Graduate Work," *Jour. Mich. St. Med. Soc.* 9 (April 1910): 186–87; "List of County Societies Following the Course of Postgraduate Study," *AMA Bulletin* 5 (15 Nov. 1909): 187–92; J. N. McCormack, "Medical Organization," *Transactions of the Tennessee State Medical Association*, 71st ann. sess. (Chattanooga, 1904), p. 61.

28. McCormack, "Things about Doctors," p. 35.

29. McCormack, "Organization of the Minnesota State Medical Association," pp. 51, 55.

30. McCormack, "The Great Work Being Done in Texas," p. 30.

31. Ibid.

32. Editorial, *Jour. Kans. Med. Soc.* 9 (April 1909): 137–38.

33. McCormack, "Things about Doctors," pp. 31–38; *Jour. Med. Soc. St. N.J.* 2 (May 1906): 349; *Wis. Med. Jour.* 8 (Oct. 1909): 274–75. Writers have generally considered Ivy L. Lee the pioneer in the field of public relations. In 1906 he attempted to improve the public image of the anthracite coal operators whose oppressive practices were exposed in the great strike of 1902. In 1912 he took over the publicity work of the Pennsylvania Railroad and shortly after was employed by the Rockefeller interests to improve their public image following the "Ludlow Massacre" of 1914. Yet his activities fell far short of McCormack's work. For accounts of Lee's career see Wayne W. Parrish, " 'Ivy Lee,' Family Physician to Big Business," *Literary Digest* 117 (9 June 1934): 30; Eric F. Goldman, *Two-Way Street: The Emergence of the Public Relations Counsel* (Boston: Bellman Pub. Co., 1948), p. 7; Stanley Kelley, Jr., *Professional Public Relations and Political Power* (Baltimore: The Johns Hopkins Press, 1956), pp. 9–38; and Alan R. Raucher, *Public Relations and Business* (Baltimore: The Johns Hopkins Press, 1968), pp. 17–31. None of these writers refers to McCormack's record.

34. McCormack, "Things about Doctors," p. 33.

35. Editorial, *Md. Med. Jour.* 50 (April 1907): 160; *Jour. Kans. Med. Soc.* 5 (1 Jan. 1905): 1, quoting an unidentified issue of *JAMA;* McCormack, "Medical Organization," p. 63.

36. McCormack, "Things about Doctors," p. 33.

37. Ibid., pp. 33–34; McCormack, "Organization and Its Advantages," p. 226.

38. McCormack, "Things about Doctors," pp. 32–33, 37, quotation, p. 36.

39. Ibid., pp. 36–37; McCormack, "The Great Work Being Done in Texas," p. 31.

40. "Annual Report of the Council," *Ill. Med. Jour.* 10 (July 1906): 57; "Report of the Board of Censors," *Transactions of the Medical Association of the State of Alabama* (Mobile, 1907), p. 71; *Ohio St. Med. Jour.* 4 (15 Dec. 1908): 730.

41. "Annual Report of the Council," *Ill. Med. Jour.* 10 (July 1906): 57; Editorial, *Ohio St. Med. Jour.* 4 (15 Dec. 1908): 730; *ibid.* 4 (15 Oct. 1908): 681.

42. "Report of the Board of Censors," *Trans. Med. Assn. St. Ala.,* 1907, p. 71.

43. *Jour. Kans. Med. Soc.* (1 Jan. 1905): 1, quoting from an unidentified issue of *JAMA.*

44. Editorial, *Ohio St. Med. Jour.* 2 (15 Dec. 1906): 310–11, 314; McCormack, "Oregon Practically An Unorganized State," p. 1818–19; Editorial, *Northwest Med.* 4 (June 1906): 205; James A. Egan and George W. Webster, correspondence with J. N. McCormack, *Ill. Med. Jour.* 11 (May 1907): 553–68, copied from *Illinois State Board of Health Bulletin,* Feb. 1907. For an example of Lydston's fight against the principal leaders of the AMA see "The Evolution of a Medical Despotism in the United States with a Few Non-Official Remedies for the Same," *New Orleans Med. Surg. Jour.* 62 (Nov. 1909): 369–85. He refers to the AMA's alleged effort to combine trust, monopoly, and trade unionism. Of McCormack, he said, "He is eloquent, persuasive, bland and suave, and can make oratory assume the fair front of argument, and like a veritable master of linguistic necromancy, transforms palpable sophistry into a veri-similitude of logic" (p. 379). See also "The Russianizing of American Medicine and the Medical Dreyfus," *Amer. Med. Compend.* 26 (Feb. 1910) 38–41. This conflict became so bitter that McCormack temporarily forgot his crusade against professional criticism and referred to Lydston, a professor of surgical diseases of the genito-urinary organs at the University of Illinois School of Medicine, as a "specialist in the filthiest of human diseases." See Editorial, *Wis. Med. Jour.* 7 (April 1909): 663, in which he is criticized for this statement.

45. *Jour. Osteop.* 16 (May 1909): 373–74, 379–81; "Report of the Committee on Organization," *JAMA* 46 (16 June 1906): 1870.

46. *JAMA* 57 (8 July 1911): 140; Burrow, *AMA,* pp. 44–45.

47. See note 33 above. Recently the outstanding public relations work of Herbert Hoover that began in 1912 has been emphasized, but his record, at least before World War I, does not at all match McCormack's work. For this part of Hoover's career see Craig Lloyd, *Aggressive Introvert: A Study of Herbert Hoover and Public Relations Management, 1912–1933* (Columbus: Ohio State University Press, 1972), esp. pp. 19–33.

48. McCormack's own training did not match the educational standards he sought to establish for the profession. Yet his success in practice, the distinction with which he served on the Kentucky state board of health, and the high ideals he held up before physicians throughout the nation symbolized the noblest aspirations of the profession (McCormack, "Some Personal Sketches," *Ky. Med. Jour.* 21 [Jan. 1923]: 20–25, and *JAMA* 78 [13 May 1922]: 1475).

CHAPTER THREE

1. George Dock, "Spelling as an Index to the Preparation of the Medical Student," *JAMA* 52 (10 April 1909): 1177; Lincoln Cothran, "Preliminary Education," *Calif. St. Jour. Med.* 3 (Sept. 1905): 281; Julius H. Comroe, "Prescribing versus Dispensing," *Pa. Med. Jour.* 12 (Oct. 1908): 22. For other examples see Editorial, *Jour. Kans. Med. Soc.* 4 (Jan. 1904): 167, which cites an unidentified issue of *Medical Fortnightly*, and Inez C. Philbrick, "Medical Colleges and Professional Standards," *JAMA* 36 (15 June 1901): 1701. Many colorful answers to examination questions are given by the National Board of Medical Examiners in *Md. Med. Jour.* 50 (July 1907): 284.

2. Editorial, *Ill. Med. Jour.* 12 (July 1907): 79. In 1906, Mervin T. Sudler, dean of the scientific department of the University of Kansas School of Medicine, remarked, "In America, be it said to our shame, we have the lowest and poorest medical standards of any of the great civilized countries." Less than ten of the nation's schools, he charged, had standards as high as the weakest of foreign universities ("The Problem of Medical Education in America," *Jour. Kans. Med. Soc.* 6 [1 Aug. 1906]: 324).

3. J. G. Dean, "The Doctor, The Public and Medical Legislation," *Transactions of the Medical Association of Georgia* (Athens, 1910), p. 67; *Ind. Med. Jour.* 20 (Dec. 1901): 216; *Ill. Med. Jour.*, n.s. 5 (Sept. 1903): 254.

4. Arthur Dean Bevan, "Cooperation in Medical Education and Medical Services," *JAMA* 90 (14 April 1928): 1175; J. A. Witherspoon, "Medical Education—Past, Present and Future," *Southern Med. Jour.* 2 (Nov. 1909): 1702. Figures on the number of medical schools in the United States in 1904 show some variation, but Bevan's number, cited here, agrees with the chart in Editorial, *JAMA* 55 (20 Aug. 1910): 695. The Reference Committee on Medical Education of the AMA in its report of 1910 set the figure at 168; N. P. Colwell, writing in 1922, set 161, and an editorial in *JAMA* in 1904 set the number at 157. See "Report of the Reference Committee on Medical Education," *JAMA* 54 (18 June 1910): 2061; N. P. Colwell, Remarks, *AMA Bulletin* 16 (15 Feb. 1922): 70; Editorial, *JAMA* 43 (13 Aug. 1904): 466. Since medical schools often opened and closed rapidly in this period the variations in numbers may result partially from information acquired at different times in the year as well as from some inaccuracies in compilation.

5. *JAMA* 42 (18 June 1904): 1646; Editorial, *JAMA* 37 (16 Nov. 1901): 1320; "Report of Committee on Medical Legislation," *JAMA* 42 (11 June 1904): 1576. The membership of the council included William T. Councilman (Mass.), with a term of one year; John A. Witherspoon (Tenn.), two years; Charles H. Frazier (Pa.), three years; Victor C. Vaughn (Mich.), four years, and Arthur D. Bevan (Ill.), five years (*JAMA* 42 [18 June 1904]: 1646). The AMA had a committee on medical education before the council was established, but its work had been largely ineffective (Editorial, *JAMA* 54 [21 May 1910]: 1694).

6. "Standards of Medical Education Adopted by the American Medical Association, July, 1905," *JAMA* 47 (25 Aug. 1906): 627.

7. *JAMA* 47 (25 Aug. 1906): 269–70; Walter Lindley, Remarks, *Calif. St. Jour. Med.* 3 (Sept. 1905): 282. The council's plan did not require college training of students before they entered medical schools. The *JAMA* had indicated in 1902 that no higher standards could be expected at the time ("Preliminary Examinations for Medical Degrees," *JAMA* 38 [Jan. 1902]: 38). The Chicago conference actually recommended a medical curriculum of four thousand hours, and for its structure see *JAMA* 45 (19 Aug. 1905): 564.

8. "Standards of Medical Education," p. 627.

9. "Report of the Council on Medical Education," *JAMA* 46 (16 June 1906): 1853; N. P. Colwell, Remarks, *JAMA* 48 (18 May 1907): 1707; Bevan, "Cooperation in Medical Education," pp. 1174–75. Committees on medical education had been established in all of the states except Alabama, Arkansas, Nevada, South Carolina, and Tennessee (Colwell, Remarks, p. 1707).

10. For the standards of the Association of American Medical Colleges and the entrance requirements of the Southern Medical Association, the American Institute of Homeopathy, and the National Confederation of Eclectic Medical Colleges see "Standards of Medical Education," pp. 627, 632–35. The AMA survived on a modest income throughout all of this period and sometimes complained that it had assumed the costs of functions properly belonging to the federal government. See James G. Burrow, *AMA: Voice of American Medicine* (Baltimore: The Johns Hopkins Press, 1963), p. 125.

11. Arthur D. Bevan, Remarks, *JAMA* 48 (18 May 1907): 1702.

12. Ibid.

13. Bevan, "Cooperation in Medical Education," p. 1175; Editorial, *JAMA* 54 (21 May 1910): 1966. In 1906, the AMA's Council on Medical Education listed Kentucky as one of the five "especially rotten spots" on the educational front. The other four states were Illinois, Maryland, Missouri, and Tennessee. See "Report of Council on Medical Education," p. 1853.

14. N. P. Colwell, Remarks, *AMA Bulletin* 16 (15 Feb. 1922): 70; Editorial, *JAMA* 54 (21 May 1910): 1695.

15. W. T. Councilman to Harvey Cushing, 4 April 1907, folder, "Correspondence: University and Hospital Appointments," Harvey Cushing File, Yale Medical Historical Library, New Haven, Conn.

16. Bevan, Remarks, p. 1702; Bevan, "Cooperation in Medical Education," pp. 1174–75. In the latter citation Bevan states that medical schools were divided into three classes based on the findings of the inspection and that all schools rating above 70 were classified as A, but this does not correspond with his report in 1907 and seems to be incorrect.

17. "Report of Committee on Medical Education," *Ill. Med. Jour.* 12 (July 1907): 62; "Report of The Texas Representative of the Council on Medical Education," *Texas St. Jour. Med.* 3 (June 1907): 77; "Report of the Texas Representative," ibid. 6 (June 1910): 41.

18. Editorial, *Jour. Mo. St. Med. Assn.* 4 (July 1907): 39–40; Editorial, ibid. 4 (Aug. 1907): 114.

19. *Pa. Med. Jour.* 15 (April 1912): 566; "Report of the Secretary of the Council on Medical Education," *JAMA* 50 (16 May 1908): 1644.

20. "Report of Secretary," p. 1645.

21. Ibid., p. 1646; Arthur D. Bevan, "Medical Education in the United States; the Need for a Uniform Standard," *JAMA* 51 (15 Aug. 1908): 570.

22. Editorial, *JAMA* 54 (21 May 1910): 1694–95. In establishing the Committee of One Hundred, the council divided the area of medical education into ten parts and appointed a chairman for each of the sections who, in turn, selected nine others to work with him. This curriculum is presented by Bevan in his remarks at the Fifth Annual Conference on Medical Education (*JAMA* 52 [8 May 1909]: 152). For additional information see J. W. Holland, Remarks, *Proceedings of the Association of American Medical Colleges, Twentieth Annual Meeting, Baltimore, March 21–22 1910* (Baltimore, 1910), pp. 55–56.

23. Bevan, "Medical Education in the United States," p. 570; "Report of the Council on Medical Education," *JAMA* 57 (1 July 1911): 82–83.

24. Bevan, "Medical Education in the United States," p. 568.

25. Ibid.

26. "Report of the Council on Medical Education," *JAMA* 54 (11 June 1910): 1974–75; "Report of the Council on Medical Education," *JAMA* 58 (8 June 1912): 1793.

27. Bevan, "Cooperation in Medical Education," p. 1175; "Report of the Council on Medical Education," *JAMA* 58 (8 June 1912): 1793. The list of colleges rated in the second inspection totaled 136. But 13 medical schools were closed in 1910; apparently 10 of these were closed after the second inspection and by the end of the year, reducing the number to 126.

28. "Report of the Council on Medical Education," *JAMA* 54 (11 June 1910): 1977–79; "Reference Committee on Medical Education," *JAMA* 54 (18 June 1910): 2061–62. For a list of the homeopathic and eclectic medical schools about 1900 see *Transactions of the American Institute of Homeopathy* 57 (Richfield Springs, N.Y.: 1901), pp. 729–33; Editorial, *Eclectic Med. Jour.* 75 (Aug. 1915): 433.

29. "Report of the Council on Medical Education," *JAMA* 54 (11 June 1910): 1974–79.

30. Bevan, "Cooperation in Medical Education," p. 1175; copy of address of Abraham Flexner, 24 Feb. 1927, Philadelphia, p. 13, "Welch Biography, Notes and Other Material Used in Preparation," Box 217, William H. Welch Papers, The Johns Hopkins Institute of the History of Medicine, Baltimore, Md.; manuscript, "The State of Medical Education Prior to the Flexner Report," p. 6, Carnegie File: General Correspondence, Box 17; and letter copy [Flexner] to C. W. Eliot, 14 June 1904, Carnegie File, Professional Education, Box 19, Abraham Flexner Papers, Manuscripts Division, Library of Congress, Washington, D.C.

31. Abraham Flexner, *An Autobiography* (New York: Simon and Shuster, 1960), pp. 74, 75, 78; quotation, Abraham Flexner, *I Remember: The Autobiography of Abraham Flexner* (New York: Simon and Shuster, 1940), p. 130. Twenty years later Flexner told Welch, "I could myself have done nothing without you—and in justice I should add, without [Franklin P.] Mall,—for from you and him I learned all that I know of medical education" (Flexner to Welch, 1 April 1930, Flexner Correspondence, Box 25, Welch Papers). Flexner said that he finished his inspection in less than one year (Flexner, *I Remember*, p. 130). In his report he gave the month in which he made his last inspection. Actually, his inspection was completed by the end of April 1910, during which month he inspected only one new school. In April he inspected the Manhattan Eye, Ear, and Throat Hospital and reinspected the Eclectic Medical Institute of Cincinnati. See Abraham Flexner, with an introduction by Henry S. Pritchett, *Medical Education in the United States and Canada: A Report of the Carnegie Foundation for the Advancement of Teaching*, Bulletin No. 4 (New York: [The Carnegie Foundation for the Advancement of Teaching], 1910, reprint, 1960), passim, and esp. pp. 263–64, 274–75, 283–84. For a recent brief treatment of this report see Martin Kaufman, *American Medical Education: The Formative Years, 1765–1910* (Westport, Conn.: The Greenwood Press, 1976), pp. 167–74.

32. Flexner, *Medical Education in the United States*, pp. 188, 205, 258.

33. Ibid., pp. 227, 191, 201–3, 217.

34. Flexner's opposition to proprietary and sectarian schools appears throughout the report and repeatedly he cites the "equivalent" abuse.

35. See copy of Writ and Petition, Circuit Court, City of St. Louis, filed by Col-

lege of Physicians and Surgeons, Carnegie File: Professional Education, Box 20; Colwell to Pritchett, 13 June 1916, and Simmons to Pritchett, 15 June 1910, Carnegie File: Professional Education, Box 18, all in Flexner Papers. Flexner apparently referred to this case when he said he was actually sued for libel for $150,000 (Flexner, *I Remember,* p. 130). If so the figure is incorrect.

36. "The Chicago Meeting of the Council and Legislative Committee of the A.M.A.," *Jour. AIH* (2 April, 1910): 247; ibid. 3 (Sept. 1910): 226; the quotation from an unidentified issue of the *Clinical Report,* a homeopathic publication, is cited in *Nat. Eclectic Med. Assn. Quar.* 2 (Sept. 1910): 62.

37. *Jour. AIH* 3 (Oct. 1910): 310; ibid. 3 (Nov. 1910): 280.

38. Editorial, *Eclectic Med. Jour.* 70 (July 1910): 377; Editorial, ibid., 71 (Feb. 1911): 101. For the AMA's struggle to secure a national health department, see Burrow, *AMA,* pp. 93–106.

39. G. W. Thompson, "President's Address," *Nat. Eclectic Med. Assn. Quar.* 2 (Sept. 1910): 30; Editorial, *Jour. Amer. Osteop. Assn.* 9 (July 1910): 502, quotation, p. 503. For an investigation that the American Osteopathic Association had made of its own schools and its citation of certain weaknesses, see "Report of the Committee on Medical Education," ibid. 9 (Sept. 1909): 29.

40. "Report of the Council on Medical Education," *Jour. Mo. St. Med. Assn.* 8 (July 1911): 35–36; Webster, Remarks, *Ill. Med. Jour.* 19 (Jan. 1911): 101; Editorial, citing Tinkham, *Nat. Eclectic Med. Assn. Quar.* 5 (June 1914): 364, quotations, West to editor of *Collier's* (undated), and Stover to Carnegie, 8 July 1909, Carnegie File: Professional Education, Box 18, Flexner Papers.

41. Quotation in Editorial, *Eclectic Med. Jour.* 74 (April 1914): p. 192, taken from an unidentified issue of the *Homeop. Recorder.*

42. Osler to Ira Remsen, pamphlet dated 1 Sept. 1911, pp. 3–4, 10–13, "Pamphlets on Full-Time for Clinicians, 1902–1932," Cushing File. Osler's report also went to the trustees, to several professors in the medical school, and to Flexner, but it was labeled "strictly confidential."

43. Letters, John D. Rockefeller, Jr., to Wallace Buttrick, 14 Feb. 1908, and Andrew Carnegie to Wallace Buttrick, 16 Sept. 1918, General Education Board File, Box 328, Series 1, subscries 2, Folder 800.2, "Andrew Carnegie, 1907–1919," Rockefeller Archive Center, Hillcrest, Pocantico Hills, North Tarrytown, N.Y.

44. Typed manuscript, p. 4, Edwin Embree File, Box 1, Accession No. 9, Folder 3, Rockefeller Archive Center. For the brutality at Ludlow see Alvin R. Sunseri, "The Ludlow Massacre: A Study of the Mis-Employment of the National Guard," *American Chronicle* 1 (Jan. 1972): 21–28. John D. Rockefeller, Jr., owned 40 percent of the stock in this sprawling enterprise.

45. *Cincinnati Enquirer,* 18 June 1914, p. 5.

46. As quoted in Editorial, *Calif. Eclectic Med. Jour.* 7 (Aug. 1914): 196.

47. Editorial, *Ohio St. Med. Jour.* 6 (15 Oct. 1910): 556. For a summary of views expressed by several other journals see Editorial, *Ill. Med. Jour.* 18 (Aug. 1910): 234–36. For the view that the *Report* would be useful in combating the economic abuses of the profession see "Report of the Committee Appointed by the Erie County Medical Society to Investigate the Division of Fees, and Its Causes and Remedies," *N.Y. St. Jour. Med.* 11 (Feb. 1911): 95–97.

48. Flexner gives the month of each inspection. The three months here referred to are April, November, and December 1909. See Flexner, *Medical Education in the United States,* passim. Very likely Flexner did not devote even seventy-eight days to these inspections, for this number includes Saturdays, which would not have been favorable days for inspection.

49. For homeopathic and eclectic contributions to therapeutics see chapter 5 below. For the deference Flexner accorded to state institutions but apparently not to many small private schools see, for example, his letter to Burton D. Myers, secretary, Indiana University School of Medicine, 19 Feb. 1910, in which he said, "I want to deal just as lightly with the defects of Indiana University as I conscientiously can, and if you will submit to me an emendation of the passages to which you object, I assure you that I will do my best to meet what you conceive to be a fair statement of conditions" (Carnegie File: Professional Education, Harvard University Folder, Box 19, Flexner Papers). See also Flexner to James H. Baker, president of the University of Colorado, 18 Feb. 1910, Carnegie File: Professional Education, University of Denver Folder, Box 18, Flexner Papers.

50. For the view that Flexner's principal success lay in encouraging private philanthropy to support medical education see Robert P. Hudson, "Abraham Flexner in Perspective: American Medical Education, 1965–1910," *Bull. Hist. Med.* 46 (Nov.–Dec. 1972): 560–61.

51. "Report of the Council on Medical Education," *JAMA* 57 (1 July 1911): 86. For a brief account of the work of the Carnegie Foundation for the Advancement of Teaching see Robert M. Lester, *Forty Years of College Giving* (New York: Charles Scribner's Sons, 1941), pp. 45–50, and for the charter of incorporation see pp. 154–57.

52. Letter, S. P. Kramer to editor, 22 July 1915, *Ohio St. Med. Jour.* 11 (Aug. 1915): 530.

53. Simon Flexner, *The Evolution and Organization of the University Clinic* (Oxford: Clarendon Press, 1939), p. 29; *Calif. St. Jour. Med.* 12 (Aug. 1914): 356. For full details of the agreement by which the General Education Board established these endowed chairs see copy of legal document dated 23 Oct. 1913, General Education Board File, Box 588, Accession No. 23, Folder 1005, Rockefeller Archive Center.

54. For the controversy that the program aroused in the Medical Department of the Johns Hopkins University see accounts of an interview of Florence R. Sabin with William H. Welch, 9 Dec. 1933, "Welch Biography: Notes and Other Material Used in Preparation," Box 217, Welch Papers. For methods of disposing of income acquired by such plans see William Darrah, *Memorandum on the School of Medicine* (New York, 13 Dec. 1919). This pamphlet appears in "Pamphlets on Full-Time for Clinicians" in Harvey Cushing File. Darrah was dean of the College of Physicians and Surgeons, Columbia University. For mild and severe criticisms of the plan by Theodore C. Janeway, the first full-time appointee at the Department of Medicine of the Johns Hopkins University, and George Dock, the first full-time appointee at the George Washington University Department of Medicine, see Philip E. Rothman, "The Full-Time Professorship in Medical Education," pp. 5–7, reprint from *California and Western Medicine* 39 (Nov. 1928).

55. George Blumer to Abraham Flexner (copy), 22 Feb. 1915, in Folder, 1914, G. Blumer—A Flexner, Re. Rath. Lab. and Hospital, George Blumer File, Yale Medical Historical Library; *JAMA* 64 (16 Jan. 1915): 257; Arthur D. Bevan, "Supplement to the Report of the Council on Medical Education and Hospitals," *JAMA* 76 (18 June 1921): 1764–66.

56. Editorial, *JAMA* 56 (8 April 1911): 1041.

57. "Report of the Council on Medical Education," *JAMA* 63 (8 June 1912): 1775, 1797–98.

58. N. P. Colwell, Remarks, *AMA Bulletin* 16 (15 Feb. 1922): 30.

59. Editorial, *New Orleans Med. Surg. Jour.* 67 (Aug. 1914): 174.

60. "State Board Statistics for 1916: Annual Presentation of the Council on Medical Education," *JAMA* 68 (14 April 1917): 1120; "Report of the Reference Committee on Medical Education," *JAMA* 66 (24 June 1916): 2083–84.

CHAPTER FOUR

1. Charles A. L. Reed, "President's Address," *JAMA* 36 (8 June 1901): 1606. For accounts of the regular profession's strategy in seeking legislative controls over the medical profession in the late nineteenth century see Donald E. Konold, *A History of American Medical Ethics, 1874–1912* (Madison: The State Historical Society of Wisconsin, 1962), pp. 28–29, and William G. Rothstein, *American Physicians in the Nineteenth Century: From Sect to Science* (Baltimore: The Johns Hopkins University Press, 1972), pp. 305–10.

2. For a brief account of some of the minor sects not treated below see Editorial, *JAMA* 43 (13 Aug. 1904): 466. For the persistence of three physiomedical schools and for the work of the American Electro-Therapeutic Association, that held its first meeting in 1891, see Francis B. Bishop, "President's Address," *Transactions of the American Electro-Therapeutic Association,* 1899 (Philadelphia: F. A. Davis Co., 1901), p. 17, and Walter H. White, "President's Address," ibid. (1901), p. 180. For comments on Dowieism, the Emmanuel Movement, and psychic systems generally see John Swain, "John Alexander Dowie; The Prophet and His Profits," *Century Magazine* 64 (Oct. 1902): 933–44; Martin J. Sweeney, "Psychic Remedies and the Irregulars," *Pa. Med. Jour.* 10 (Sept. 1907): 951; Editorial, *N.Y. Med. Jour.* 87 (30 May 1908): 1047–48; Lyman P. Powell, "What Is the Emmanuel Movement?" *Ladies Home Journal* 25 (Nov. 1908): 7–8, and ibid. 26 (Dec. 1908): 9. For a recent treatment see Donald Meyer, *The Positive Thinkers: A Study of the American Quest For Health, Wealth and Personal Power from Mary Baker Eddy to Norman Vincent Peale* (Anchor Books, New York: Doubleday & Co., 1966), pp. 231–32, 237–38.

3. Meyer, *Positive Thinkers,* p. 20.

4. Andrew T. Still, "How I Came to Originate Osteopathy," *Ladies Home Journal* 25 (Jan. 1908): 25; C. M. Turner Hulett, "Address," *Jour. Amer. Osteop. Assn.* 9 (April 1910): 353; C. M. Turner Hulett, "Historical Sketch of the AAAO," ibid. 1 (Sept. 1901): 1. Still traced the origins of osteopathy to 1874, but indicated that his views had been developed much earlier. "I began to give reasons," he said, "for my faith in the laws of life as given by men, worlds, and beings by the God of nature, in April, 1855" (*The Philosophy and Mechanical Principles of Osteopathy* [Kansas City: Hudson-Kimberley Pub. Co., 1902], p. 9); E. R. Booth, *History of Osteopathy and Twentieth-Century Medical Practice* (Cincinnati: Caxton Press, 1905, rev. 1924), pp. 86–88, and for other schools started before 1900 see pp. 88–93.

5. Hulett, "Historical Sketch," pp. 1–2, 19. The American Osteopathic Association was called the American Association for the Advancement of Osteopathy when it was established 19 April 1897.

6. Still, *Philosophy and Principles of Osteopathy,* p. 9.

7. Ibid., p. 18.

8. *Osteopathy As Taught by Dr. A. T. Still and the American School of Osteopathy* (Kirksville, Mo.: The American School of Osteopathy), A. T. Still File, "Osteopathic Pictures, Historical," Library of the Kirksville College of Osteopathy and Surgery, Kirksville, Mo.; M. Clayton Thrush, "Osteopathic versus Drug Treatment," *JAMA* 51 (19 Dec. 1908): 2137; quotations, "Our Platform," *Jour. Osteop.* 9 (Oct. 1902): 342.

9. Andrew T. Still, *Philosophy of Osteopathy* (Kirksville, Mo.: A. T. Still, 1899), p. 208.

10. Louis S. Reed, *The Healing Cults: A Study of Sectarian Medical Practice: Its Extent, Causes, and Control*, The Committee on the Costs of Medical Care, Publication No. 16 (Chicago: University of Chicago Press, 1932), pp. 107–8; Stanford Research Institute, Southern California Laboratories, *Chiropractic in California: A Report* (Los Angeles: Hayes Foundation, 1960), p. 14; *Chiropractor's Adjuster* (1910), p. 11, cited in Theodore Schreiber, "The Fundamental Basis for All Scientific Research," *Nat. Chirop.* 16 (Dec. 1946): 31.

11. Leslie Brainerd Arey et al., eds., *Dorland's Illustrated Medical Dictionary*, 23d ed. (Philadelphia: W. B. Saunders Co., 1957), pp. 1069, 300. For quotation from Hunter and his fuller description see "Chiropractic Adequately Considered Weighed in the Balance and Found Out," *Jour. Osteop.* 16 (Feb. 1909): 72. Osteopaths and chiropractors both claimed that their rival had borrowed the other's techniques. Hunter maintained that chiropractic was "mutilated osteopathy" and that it confined itself to a "subdivision of osteopathy" (ibid. pp. 71–72). For the claim that osteopaths had borrowed chiropractic methods see Joy M. Laban, *Technic and Practice of Chiropractic*, 3d rev. ed. (Pittsburgh: Laban Pub. Co., 1918), p. 401.

12. Stanford Research Institute, *Chiropractic in California*, p. 91.

13. Ibid., pp. 14, 1, 15.

14. James Thorington, "Refracting Opticians," *Pa. Med. Jour.* 13 (Feb. 1910): 369; "Resolution Adopted by the Peoria City Medical Society, Dec. 20, 1910," *Ill. Med. Jour.* 19 (Jan. 1911): 125; J. W. Charles, "Why Physicians Should Actively Fight the Optometry Bill," *Jour. Mo. St. Med. Assn.* 9 (Dec. 1912): 183–85.

15. Editorial, *Ohio St. Med. Jour.* 7 (15 March 1911): 134; quotation, David R. Silver, "President's Address," ibid. 5 (15 June 1909): 343.

16. *Texas St. Jour. Med.* 10 (March 1915): 477; Leartus Conner, "Family Physician Refracting as a Factor in Medical Practice, and Its Practice in 1910," *Jour. Mich. St. Med. Soc.* 9 (Oct. 1910): 551; James Thorington, "The Prescribing of Glasses by the Family Physician," *Pa. Med. Jour.* 15 (1 July 1912): 777. In 1910 another physician, Albert R. Baker, criticized the proposed medical curriculum of the Council on Medical Education for allowing only 50 hours out of a total of 4,478 to training in eye refraction "Teaching Ophthalmology," (*Proceedings of the Twentieth Annual Meeting of the Association of American Medical Colleges* [Baltimore, 1910], pp. 88–89).

17. See the *Sun* (New York), 16 Dec. 1898, p. 6, for Mrs. Eddy's claim, and the *Sun*, 1 Jan. 1899, p. 6, for Reed's challenge.

18. Thos. F. Duhigg, "Where Chiropractors Are Made," *Texas St. Jour. Med.* 12 (Dec. 1916): 364–65, reprint from the *West Virginia Medical Journal*, Dec. 1916. Duhigg based his case on findings of the Pennsylvania Bureau of Medical Education and Licensure.

19. The profession, of course, favored reciprocity laws that would make concessions to thoroughly qualified physicians who wished to move beyond their state to practice and who saw no need for taking licensing examinations elsewhere.

20. William Duffield, "Some Observations on Medical Legislation," *Colo. Med. Jour.. and Western Gaz.* 7 (Feb. 1901): 59–61. These states and territories were, along with the District of Columbia, Alabama, Arizona, Connecticut, Delaware, Florida, Georgia, Idaho, Illinois, Indian Territory, Iowa, Louisiana, Missouri, Maryland, Massachusetts, Minnesota, New Hampshire, New Jersey, New York, North Carolina, North Dakota, Ohio, Oregon, Pennsylvania, South Carolina, Tennessee,

Texas, Utah, Virginia, Washington, West Virginia, and Wisconsin. Duffield strangely omits Alabama which here is included.

21. A. S. Burdick, "Some Phases of Medical Practice Legislation," *Ill. Med. Jour.* 3 (July 1901): 60–61; "Medical Practice Laws," *AMA Bulletin* 3 (15 Nov. 1907): 36, 41.

22. "Medical Practice Laws," p. 37; *JAMA* 50 (16 May 1908): 1643.

23. Statistics on the structure of state medical boards and other of their characteristics are based on an analysis of state medical practice laws as they appear under the heading of the states in *Amer. Med. Dir.*, 6th ed. (Chicago: American Medical Association, 1918). The five states with multiple boards were Arkansas, Delaware, Florida, Louisiana, and Maryland.

24. The states requiring that appointments to the board be made from a list recommended by the state societies were Alabama, Connecticut, Delaware, Kentucky, Louisiana, Michigan, Pennsylvania, South Carolina, Vermont, Virginia, and Wisconsin. The fourteen states that allowed no system to have a majority on the board were Arizona, Georgia, Idaho, Indiana, Kansas, Massachusetts, Michigan, Nebraska, Ohio, Oklahoma, Oregon, Texas, Vermont, and Wisconsin.

25. See Chapter 5 for an account of the decline of the homeopathic and eclectic movements.

26. *Amer. Med. Dir.*, 1918, p. 727. For a long time in Greater New York an osteopath could not sign a transit permit for removing a body even if he had signed the death certificate. The legislature of Ohio did not remove the prohibition that osteopaths could not use anesthetics and antiseptics until March 1917, and similar prohibitions remained in Pennsylvania until about that time. In 1918 the attorney general of Nebraska interpreted the osteopathic law of 1909 so as to prevent osteopaths from giving anesthesia in surgical or obstetrical cases except in the presence of a doctor of medicine (Booth, *History of Osteopathy*, pp. 591, 594, 598–99, 589).

27. "Report of Secretary–Treasurer," *Twentieth Ann. Meeting Assn. Amer. Med. Coll.*, p. 113; Booth, *History of Osteopathy*, pp. 102–61, 562–612. The regular profession had reason to fear the efforts of osteopaths to secure separate boards after they got their board in California in 1901. Within five years their board granted 490 licenses upon the basis of diplomas and without examinations (Dudley Tait, "Work of the Board of Medical Examiners," *Calif. St. Jour. Med.* 4 [Nov. 1906]: 286). Beverly D. Harrison, chairman of the AMA's committee responsible for drafting a model medical practice act, said that in six years after the osteopaths in California secured their independent board they issued 900 licenses. See F. E. Moore, "Read, Think and Act," *Jour. Amer. Osteop. Assn.* 8 (Dec. 1908): 174.

28. Editorial, *Del. St. Med. Jour.* 2 (March 1930): 51; Julius Dintenfass, *Chiropractic: A Modern Way to Health* (New York: Pyramid Books, 1965), pp. 162–67; *Outlook* 114 (1 Nov. 1916): 483; Committee on Optometry Legislation, "A Statement Concerning the 'Optometry Bill' and 'Optometrists,' " *Jour. Mo. St. Med. Assn.* 7 (Feb. 1911): 277; James R. Gregg, *American Optometric Association: A History* (St. Louis: American Optometric Association, 1972), pp. 365–66.

29. The regular medical profession was seeking legal support in its drive for higher educational standards and made effective use of the law for this purpose during this era.

30. By 1917 the laws of five states specifically required the standards set by the American or Southern associations, or standards just as high for institutions whose graduates would be allowed to take the licensing examinations. These states were Arizona, Maryland, Missouri, Oklahoma, and Washington. For these laws see *Amer. Med. Dir.*, 1918, pp. 202, 699, 973, 1290, 1611.

31. Ibid., 5th ed., 1916, p. 223; ibid., 1918, p. 1511. In 1905 twenty-seven states

required that an institution must be "reputable," "approved by the board," or "in good standing." Twenty-eight states had adopted this requirement twelve years later and three others had close approximations ("Medical Practice Laws," p. 64 and *Amer. Med. Dir.*, 1918, passim). The medical boards often interpreted these requirements to mean that the standards of the colleges must equal those set by one of the accrediting associations. Such interpretations held weight in court when a board had to defend its assessment of a particular school.

32. "Report of the Board of Trustees," *JAMA* 54 (11 June 1910): 1971; "Medical Practice Laws," p. 72; *Amer. Med. Dir.*, 1918, p. 1212.

33. "Abstract of State Osteopathic Requirements," *Jour. Osteop.* 22 (April 1915): 213, 215.

34. "Report of the Board of Trustees," p. 1971; "Medical Practice Laws," pp. 51, 52, 57. The nine states giving no definition of medical practice were California, Florida, Massachusetts, Mississippi, Missouri, New Hampshire, North Carolina, North Dakota, and Pennsylvania. The AMA never adopted the definition of medical practice that its committee drew up, nor did it offer an acceptable model medical practice bill to its membership; it struggled with the problem long after the Progressive Era closed. See, for example, *Proceedings of the House of Delegates of the American Medical Association,* 76th ann. sess. (Atlantic City, May 1925), p. 17.

35. "Medical Practice Laws," p. 56. In 1902 a prominent writer on medical jurisprudence, Henry Beates, Jr., proposed a definition of medical practice superior to that of any law for its brevity and comprehensiveness. The practice of medicine was "for any one, except those carrying out the directions of the attending physician, to engage directly or indirectly, habitually or occasionally, in the care, management or treatment, by any means whatsoever, either material or immaterial, for the relief or cure of any or all diseases, accidents, or disabilities to which human or animal life is exposed, threatened, or afflicted" ("How Should the Practice of Medicine Be Legally Defined?" *Bull. Amer. Acad. Med.* 5 (June 1902): 845–46.

36. For a variety of exceptions tolerated by the medical profession in medical practice laws see "Medical Practice Laws," p. 94, and for its emphasis on the incapacity of drugless practitioners to diagnose disease see Emil Amberg, Communication, *Jour. Mich. St. Med. Soc.* 2 (April 1903): 178.

37. "Report of Board of Trustees," p. 1971.

38. James G. Burrow, *AMA: Voice of American Medicine* (Baltimore: The Johns Hopkins Press, 1963), p. 33.

39. "Medical Practice Laws," pp. 52, 57. *Amer. Med. Dir.*, 1918, pp. 209, 374, 603, 978, 1333, 1452, 1584, 1612. These ten states were Arkansas, Florida, Georgia, Kansas, Mississippi, New Hampshire, Pennsylvania, South Carolina, Virginia, and Washington. In 1917, Florida and Mississippi still had provided no grounds for the revocation of licenses (see ibid., pp. 360, 865).

40. "Medical Practice Laws," pp. 80, 81; *Amer. Med. Dir.*, 1916, p. 225; ibid., 1918, p. 565.

41. "Medical Practice Laws," pp. 86–87; *Amer. Med. Dir.*, 1918, pp. 210, 225, 406, 565, 603, 788, 885, 1176, 1291, 1316, 1468. In 1907 the three states were Idaho, Michigan, and Oregon; those added a decade later were Arkansas, California, Iowa, Kansas, Ohio, Oklahoma, and South Dakota.

42. *Amer. Med. Dir.*, 1918, pp. 565–66, 602–3, 787–89, 1213, 1467–68, 301. These five states were Iowa, Kansas, Michigan, Ohio, and South Dakota.

43. "Medical Reciprocity," *JAMA* 34 (19 May 1900): 1666–67; Editorial, *JAMA* 37 (7 June 1902): 1524–26; William L. Rodman, "A Voluntary Board of Medical Examiners," *JAMA* 38 (10 May 1902): 1215; Editorial, ibid., p. 1233.

44. "Report of Committee on Legislation," *Jour. Mich. St. Med. Soc.* 1 (Sept.

1902): 88; James A. Egan to editor, *Ill. Med. Jour.* 12 (July 1907): 82.

45. William L. Rodman, "Work of the American Medical Association," *JAMA* 64 (26 June 1915): 2113; James N. Baker, Remarks, *Transactions of the Medical Association of the State of Alabama* (Mobile, 1916), pp. 171–72; "Report of the Council on Medical Education," *JAMA* 70 (15 June 1918): 1846. Medical leaders knew that no national licensing board was possible. J. C. Mahr, Oklahoma's state commissioner of health, said in 1914 that, "though such a law might be desirable as a practical fact, it is at present impossible for the single reason that Congress has no power to pass such an act" (*Jour. Okla. Med. Assn.* 7 [Aug. 1914]: 83).

46. In 1914 the AMA published a digest of six hundred Supreme Court decisions on state regulations of medical practice, some of which are cited below. In 1922, Frederick R. Green, secretary of the AMA's Council on Health and Public Instruction, stated that the Supreme Court had made about eight thousand decisions on medical practice (Remarks, *AMA Bulletin* 16 [15 Feb. 1922]: 35).

47. American Medical Association, Medico-Legal Bureau, comp., *A Digest of the Case Law on the Statutory Regulation of the Practice of Medicine* (Chicago: American Medical Association, 1915), p. 341.

48. Ibid., pp. 255–56; "Supreme Court Sustains the State Medical Law," *Calif. St. Jour. Med.* 2 (July 1904): 209–11. For a summary of the general conclusions on medical practice laws reached by the United States Supreme Court and the supreme courts of the states see Frederick R. Green, *State Regulation of the Practice of Medicine* (Chicago: American Medical Association, 1917), p. 14.

49. Dent. v. State of West Virginia, 129 U.S. *Supreme Court Reports,* 624 (1888). Cases in which the courts upheld the right to apply the standards of the Association of American Medical Colleges or of a comparable body to medical schools include Illinois State Board of Health v. The People, 102 Ill. App. 614 (1902); Ex parte Gerino, 77 Pac. 166 (1904); and Arwine v. Board of Medical Examiners of California, 91 Pac. 319 (1907). See AMA, *Digest of Case Law,* pp. 289–90, 256, 258.

50. Reetz v. Michigan, 188 U.S. *Supreme Court Reports,* 566 (1902).

51. Raaf v. State Board of Medical Examiners, 84 Pac. 33 (1906), and quoted in AMA, *Digest of Case Law,* p. 278. The significance of this decision is partially indicated by the fact that Montana's medical practice law allowed applicants who had failed the medical examination to secure a trial before a lay jury in a district court that would decide on their qualifications (Charles McIntire, "State Requirements for the Practice of Medicine: Revision for 1898," *Bull. Amer. Acad. Med.* 3 [Feb. 1899]: 634).

52. Roy Lubove, *The Struggle for Social Security, 1900–1935* (Cambridge: Harvard University Press, 1968), p. 89.

53. C. C. Teall, Remarks, *Jour. Amer. Osteop. Assn.* 1 (March 1902): 167.

54. Ibid. 5 (April 1906): 341; Charles Hazzard, Remarks, ibid. 5 (June 1906): 429.

55. Booth, *History of Osteopathy,* p. 149.

56. Charles W. Little, Remarks, *Jour. Osteop.* 8 (July 1901): 226.

57. *Transactions of the Medical Association of the State of Alabama* (Mobile, 1903), pp. 15, 16, 72–73; Samuel Wallace Weld, "Monitor's Address," ibid. (Birmingham, 1912), p. 175; G. Ligon, Report, *Jour. Osteop.* 13 (Sept. 1906): 267–77. For a far different bill dealing with osteopathy approved 26 Feb. 1903, see *Trans. Med. Assn. St. Ala.,* 1903, pp. 99–100.

58. Editorial, *Jour. Kans. Med. Soc.* 12 (Nov. 1912): 435–36, and for comments of other medical leaders see pp. 436–42. See also Editorial, ibid. 13 (May 1913): 213; Editorial, ibid. 14 (Oct. 1914): 377–90, quotation, p. 378.

59. *Jour. Amer. Osteop. Assn.* 11 (Dec. 1911): 838; Burrow, *AMA,* pp. 100–103; *Wis. Med. Jour.* 10 (March 1912): 599, citing an item in an unidentified newspaper.

CHAPTER FIVE

1. "Echoes from the Washington Meeting," *Amer. Med. Monthly* 18 (July 1900): 143–45; *Transactions of the American Institute of Homeopathy* 56 (Washington, D.C., 1900), pp. 103–4, quotation, p. 110 (hereafter cited *Trans. AIH*). For the complete "Ode to Hahnemann" see pp. 108–12. In this volume "homeopathy" is the spelling always used to designate this sect even in the title of articles in which "homoeopathy" occasionally appears.

2. Joseph F. Kett, *The Foundation of the American Medical Profession: The Role of Institutions, 1789–1860* (New Haven: Yale University Press, 1968), pp. 135, 137; A. B. Norton, "Homeopathy in the Twentieth Century," *Trans. AIH* 57 (Richfield Springs, N.Y., 1901): 658–62, 729–33.

3. For unfavorable contrasts between homeopathy and orthodox medicine in the late nineteenth century offered by regular physicians see J. L. Ziegler, "Points of Dissimilarity between Us and Homeopathic Physicians," and Solomon Solis-Cohen, "The Dissimilarity between Physicians and Homeopathists," *JAMA* 21 (21 Oct. 1893): 615–19. For change of the motto, *similia similibus curentus* to *similia similibus curentur,* see G. B. Peck, "Homeopathy in the United States," *Hahne. Monthly* 35 (Sept. 1900): 566, and Albert Wanstall, "The Status of Homeopathy," ibid. 37 (March 1902): 163.

4. Charles H. Higgins, "The Homeopathy of Hahnemann Compared with the Homeopathy of Today," *Ohio St. Med. Jour.* 4 (15 July 1908): 408; *Ind. Med. Jour.* 20 (Feb. 1902): 319; Editorial, ibid. 20 (Sept. 1901): 107, 109. For Pratt's procedures see B. E. Dawson, comp. and ed., with an introduction by E. H. Pratt, *Orificial Surgery: Its Philosophy, Application and Technique* (Newark, N.J.: Physicians Drug News Co., 1912).

5. Geo. B. Peck, paper, *Trans. AIH,* 1900, p. 36.

6. Ibid., 1901, pp. 658–62, statistical data compiled by Thos. Franklin Smith. The actual number of homeopaths in the United States in 1900 was unknown. G. B. Peck cited an estimate of R. L. Polk & Co. in its *Medical and Surgical Register of the United States and Canada,* 5th ed. (1898) that there were "not less than 9,369 homeopaths in the United States" (Geo. B. Peck, "Homeopathy in the United States," *Hahne Monthly* 35 [Sept. 1900]: 560).

7. For the AMA's reorganizational efforts see James G. Burrow, *AMA: Voice of American Medicine* (Baltimore: The Johns Hopkins Press, 1963), pp. 27–32, 36–44, and for the establishment of its political connections see chapter 3 of that volume and chapter 4 above.

8. A. B. Norton, "Homeopathy in the Twentieth Century," *Trans. AIH,* 1901, p. 54. Norton quotes here from the presidential address of Seldon H. Talcott at the AIH session of 1889.

9. W. J. Hawkes, Remarks, *Jour. AIH* 3 (Feb. 1911): 637; Henry E. Beebe, Remarks, ibid. 4 (Dec. 1911): 625; Sanford Burton Hooker, "A Criticism and a Reply to the Two Recent Attacks upon Homeopathy," *N.E. Med. Gaz.* 49 (March 1914): 132.

10. Donald E. Konold, *A History of American Medical Ethics, 1847–1912* (Madison: The State Historical Society of Wisconsin, 1962), pp. 68–69; *Pa. Med. Jour.* 10 (Nov. 1906): 113. For membership restrictions in new state society constitutions see, for example, constitution, *Jour. Kans. Med. Soc. and Wichita Med. Jour.* 4 (1 Feb. 1904): 216, and editorial remarks, ibid. 5 (1 May 1905): 222–23.

11. Editorial, *Wis. Med. Jour.* 3 (Oct. 1904): 407; William Osler, *Aequanamitas with Other Essays to Medical Students, Nurses, and Practitioners of Medicine,* 3d ed. (Philadelphia: Blakiston Co., 1932), pp. 434–35; Milton J. Bleim to editor, *Texas St. Jour. Med.* 1 (Jan. 1906): 247.

12. Editorial, *Hahne. Monthly* 42 (Nov. 1907): 855–61.

13. H. E. Beebe, "The Attitude of the Profession—How to Correct the Indifference of Homeopathic Physicians and Its Effects," *Trans. AIH,* 63 (Norfolk, 1907): 198.

14. Frank Billings, "Medical Education in the United States," *JAMA* 40 (9 May 1903): 1273; Torald Sollman, "The Broader Aims of the Council on Pharmacy and Chemistry," *JAMA* 50 (4 April 1908): 1134; undated letter, Committee of the American Institute of Homeopathy to Contact the AMA to the President and Secretary of the American Medical Association, *Jour. AIH* 5 (June 1913): 1352, quotation, p. 1353; F. W. Parham, "Superstitions, Fads, Fetishes and Facts: A Retrospect and Forecast; the Lines on Which the Progress of the Future Must Be Worked Out," *Transactions of the Louisiana State Medical Society,* 22d ann. sess. (New Orleans, 1901), p. 72; quotation, Thomas Duke Parke, "Monitor's Address," *Transactions of the Medical Association of the State of Alabama* (Mobile, 1904), p. 187. Homeopaths traced much of professional disbelief in the efficacy of drugs to William Osler who said, "He is the best physician who knows the worthlessness of most medicines." One homeopath referred to *"Osler's black, hopeless, helpless, therapeutic pessimism"* (J. H. M'Clelland, "Commencement Address," *Hahne. Monthly* 45 [Aug. 1910]: 564).

15. *New Orleans Med. Surg. Jour.* 48 (Sept. 1913): 496; quotations, letter, Committee of AIH to President and Secretary of AMA, p. 1352. For the establishment of the council and the laboratory see George H. Simmons, "Address," *JAMA* 48 (18 May 1907): 1646.

16. "Report of the Committee on the Formation of a National Association for Clinical Research," *Jour. AIH* 3 (Oct. 1910): 291. For an effort instituted in 1910 to improve the homeopathic materia medica see Howard P. Bellows, "An Address on the Movement to Reprove the Homeopathic Materia Medica," *Hahne. Monthly* 38 (June 1903): 423, 427–29, and for principal homeopathic remedies see Editorial, *Amer. Homeop.* 27 (1 Oct. 1901): 305.

17. "Editorial, *Amer. Homeop.,* p. 305; Editorial, *Jour. AIH* 4 (Aug. 1911): 196. For homeopathic skepticism of the laboratory procedures of the Council on Pharmacy and Chemistry, see editorial, *Med. Century* 18 (Feb. 1911): 58.

18. Herbert D. Schenck, Remarks, *Jour. AIH* 5 (Sept. 1912): 271, 272; "Report of the Committee on Conference with the American Medical Association," *N.E. Med. Gaz.* 48 (Sept. 1913): 496–99.

19. "Report of Committee on Conference with AMA," pp. 496–97; James G. Burrow, "Prescription-Drug Policies of the American Medical Association in the Progressive Era," in John B. Blake, ed., *Safeguarding the Public* (Baltimore: The Johns Hopkins Press, 1970), pp, 112–14, 120.

20. Editorial, *Hahne. Monthly* 48 (Feb. 1913): 136; Editorial, *Eclectic Med. Jour.* 71 (April 1911): 206; J. MacKenzie, "On the Teaching of Clinical Medicine," *British Med. Jour.,* 3 Jan. 1914, p. 20.

21. Alexander Craig to Herbert D. Schenck, 3 July 1914, *Jour. AIH* 7 (Sept. 1914): 314; "Special Report of the Work of the Council on Pharmacy and Chemistry," *JAMA* 65 (3 July 1915): 67.

22. For features of the original health department bill see Burrow, *AMA,* pp. 33–36, 93–106.

23. "Homeopathy: The Science," *Jour. AIH* 5 (Dec. 1912): 513–19, final quotation, p. 512.

24. Hugo R. Arndt, "The History of the American Institute of Homeopathy in Perfecting a Systematic Development of the Homeopathic Organization," *Trans. AIH* 63 (Norfolk, 1907): 216–26; Joseph P. Cobb, "The Necessity for Perfecting Systematic Development of the Homeopathic Organization," ibid., p. 206. The editor of the new journal was Willis A. Dewey, and one of the five members of the Journal Committee was Royal S. Copeland (Editorial, *Jour. AIH* 1 [Jan. 1909]: 36).

25. *Jour. AIH* 3 (Oct. 1910): 283–85; ibid. 3 (Jan. 1911): 538; Editorial, ibid. 3 (March 1911): 745; H. R. Arndt, leaflet reprints, ibid. 4 (Nov. 1911): 612–13; Editorial, ibid. 5 (March 1913): 1010; Pinkerton Crutcher, "Homeopathy in the Realm of Legislation," ibid. 4 (Dec. 1911): 621.

26. H. R. Arndt, Report, ibid. 3 (Nov. 1910): 272–76, quotation, p. 276; H. R. Arndt, "Address and Report," ibid. 4 (Sept. 1911): 332.

27. "Report of the Field Secretary to the Board of Trustees," ibid. 4 (Jan. 1912): 916; H. R. Arndt, Report, ibid. 4 (April 1912): 313–15.

28. "Field Secretary's Report," ibid. 5 (Aug. 1912): 169; ibid. 5 (July 1912): 64.

29. Ibid. 5 (Dec. 1912): 661; ibid. 5 (Feb. 1913): 862.

30. W. A. Dewey, "The Council on Medical Education of the AIH," *Homeop. Recorder* 28 (15 May 1913): 208–9; ibid. 29 (15 March 1914): 110.

31. W. J. Hawkes, "Causes Retarding the Spread of Homeopathy," *Jour. AIH* 5 (Nov. 1912): 530–31, 532.

32. H. C. Smith, "Concerning a Coalition of Homeopaths and Eclectics," *Pa. Med. Jour.* 19 (Feb. 1916): 370; Editorial, *Homeop. Recorder* 31 (15 Aug. 1916): 366.

33. Copeland, "Publicity for the Purpose of Educating the Intelligent Public Including the Homeopathic Profession," *Jour. AIH* 9 (April 1917): 1262, 1281; Editorial, ibid. 9 (May 1917): 1339. Although Copeland indicated that returning homeopaths would be impressed by fine laboratories and buildings, his assuring words could hardly conceal the decline of the system.

34. Martin, Kaufman, *Homeopathy in America: The Rise and Fall of A Medical Heresy* (Baltimore: The Johns Hopkins Press, 1971), pp. 166, 171. The two schools that survived were the New York Homeopathic Medical College and the Hahnemann Medical College of Philadelphia.

35. *Eclectic Med. Jour.* 68 (Jan. 1908): 53–54; H. W. Felter, "Pathfinders," *Nat. Eclectic Med. Assn. Quar.* 1 (Dec. 1909): 91; Burrow, *AMA*, p. 3.

36. *Eclectic Med. Jour.* 68 (Jan. 1908): 54. The chart from which these statistics were derived originally appeared in an unidentified issue of the *Eclectic Med. Gleaner*.

37. John K. Scudder, survey, *Nat. Eclectic Med. Assn. Quar.* 14 (March 1923): 224–25; *Eclectic Med. Jour.* 69 (June 1910): 316; ibid. 66 (Aug. 1906): 398. The Lloyd brothers, who were affiliated with the institute, prepared and sold drugs to physicians and answered countless letters requesting information. See letterhead of letter, John Uri Lloyd to Charles T. Greve, 3 Feb. 1905, J. U. Lloyd Letter Collection, Cincinnati Historical Society Library, Cincinnati, Ohio; Editorial, *Eclectic Med. Jour.* 66 (Oct. 1906): 508; J. A. Munk, "A Potent Factor of Eclecticism," *L. A. Jour. Eclectic Med.* 4 (April 1907): 104–7.

38. A. R. Collins, "Principles, Practice and Progress of the Eclectic School of Medicine," *Nat. Eclectic Med. Assn. Quar.* 7 (March 1916): 274; Editorial, *Eclectic*

Med. Jour 67 (July 1907): 384; A. F. Stephens, "Bedside vs. Laboratory," ibid. 69 (Oct. 1909): 569, quotation, p. 570.

39. John Uri Lloyd, "Our School of Medicine," *Eclectic Med. Jour.* 63 (May 1903): 238; A. F. Stephens in Editorial, ibid. 67 (Jan. 1907): 55; last quotation, Editorial, ibid. 67 (July 1907): 383. For the view that eclectic medicine was not sectarian see Collins, "Principles of the Eclectic School of Medicine," p. 275.

40. John King, Remarks, *Eclectic Med. Jour.* 44 (Nov. 1884): 528. See also quotation from editorial in *Medical Mercury* (April 1907) in *Eclectic Med. Jour.* 67 (May 1907): 304.

41. Letter, C. A. L. Reed to Editor of *Lancet-Clinic*, 7 July 1902, cited in *Eclectic News* 8 (Aug. 1902): 511.

42. Editorial, *Eclectic Med. Jour.* 67 (June 1907): 314–15.

43. Editorial, *Eclectic News* 13 (Aug. 1902): 512.

44. Herbert T. Webster, "The Merger Proposition," *Eclectic Med. Jour.* 66 (July 1906): 323; John K. Scudder, "President's Address," *Nat. Eclectic Med. Assn. Quar.* 1 (Sept. 1909): 23–24.

45. Editorial, *Eclectic Med. Jour.* 67 (Sept. 1907): 498–99; *Nat. Eclectic Med. Assn. Quar.* 2 (Sept. 1910): 14–15.

46. Editorial, *Eclectic Med. Jour.* 66 (Oct. 1906): 508.

47. Editorial, *Eclectic Med. Gleaner* 11 (March 1900): 73; letter, R. L. Thomas to W. A. Puckner, 8 Feb. 1910, *Eclectic Med. Jour.* 70 (March 1910): 158.

48. Editorial, *L. A. Jour. Eclectic Med.* 5 (Feb. 1908): 50–51; W. K. Mock, "The Necessity for Organization," *Eclectic Med. Jour.* 67 (April 1907): 178–79. For modifications in the Ohio plan by 1911 see J. A. Munk, "Open Letter to Eclectics," *Nat. Eclectic Med. Assn. Quar.* 2 (March 1911): 264–65, listing five state chairmen in Ohio.

49. George W. Thompson, Remarks, *Nat. Eclectic Med. Assn. Quar.* 1 (Sept. 1909): 69.

50. Editorial, *Jour. AIH* 1 (Nov. 1909): 540; "Recording Secretary's Report," *Nat. Eclectic Med. Assn. Quar.* 2 (Sept. 1910): 5–6; *Transactions of the National Eclectic Medical Association of the United States* (Atlantic City, N.J., 1900), pp. 386–97. A list of members totaling 442 is given in the *Transactions*.

51. Letter, Edward J. Farnum to members of the Illinois State Eclectic Medical Society, 20 Sept. 1910, in *Eclectic Med. Jour.* 70 (Oct. 1910): 488. For examples of the frequent claims of eclectics that demand for them far exceeded supply see editorial, ibid. 62 (March 1902): 167–68; Walter S. Bogart, "Eclectic Opportunities," ibid. 66 (May 1906): 212–14; Editorial, ibid. 66 (Sept. 1906): 446–47; John Uri Lloyd, Address, *Eclectic Rev.* 10 (15 May 1907): 131.

52. "Report of Chairman of the Committee on Organization," *Nat. Eclectic Med. Assn. Quar.* 5 (Sept. 1913): 7, 8, quotation, p. 6.

53. Editorial, *Eclectic Med. Jour.* 75 (Aug. 1915): 433. The other schools with their closing dates are as follows: Eclectic Medical College or College of Physicians and Surgeons, Indianapolis, 1903; Bennett College of Eclectic Medicine and Surgery, Chicago, 1909; American Medical College, St. Louis, 1910; Eclectic Medical College of the City of New York, 1913; Eclectic Medical University, Kansas City, 1914; California Medical College, Los Angeles, 1915. See John K. Scudder, compilation, *Nat. Eclectic Med. Assn. Quar.* 14 (March 1923): 224–25.

54. "Report of the Committee on Organization," *Nat. Eclectic Med. Assn. Quar.* 8 (Sept. 1916): 12, 26; Editorial, *Eclectic Med. Jour.* 75 (Aug. 1915): 434, 435.

CHAPTER SIX

1. Charles A. L. Reed, "The Medical Inspection of Schools and Medical Freedom," *Journal of Proceedings and Addresses of the National Education Association of the United States,* 50th Annual Meeting (Chicago, 1912), p. 276.

2. Editorial, *New Orleans Med. Surg. Jour.* 67 (Oct. 1914): 381. For a treatment of some of the social reforms of the early twentieth century in which some physicians took an interest see Lloyd C. Taylor, Jr., *The Medical Profession and Social Reform, 1885–1945* (New York: St. Martin's Press, 1974), pp. 1–101.

3. "Things Original from the Kansas State Board of Health," *Jour. Kans. Med. Soc.* 13 (Jan. 1913): 75–76; Thomas Neville Bonner, *The Kansas Doctor* (Lawrence: University of Kansas Press, 1959), pp. 78, 80–81, 118, and for an extensive treatment of Crumbine's work see pp. 120–71.

4. "Things Original," pp. 75–76; Bonner, *Kansas Doctor,* pp. 143, 154, 155, 144–45.

5. Albert Woldert, "A Review of State Health Departments and a Plan for a State Board of Health in Texas," *Texas St. Jour. Med.* 1 (Dec. 1905): 191, 192.

6. *Ill. Med. Jour.* 8 (July 1905): 77; H. R. M. Harris, "The Tuberculosis Crusade," *Pa. Med. Jour.* 18 (Nov. 1913): 103.

7. "Report of the Committee on Hygiene," *Transactions of the Medical Society of the State of New York* (Albany, 1900), pp. 41, 82–83; "Report of the Committee on Hygiene," ibid. (Albany, 1901), p. 24; Editorial, *Jour. Mich. St. Med. Soc.* 7 (Dec. 1908): 628; Harris, "Tuberculosis Crusade," p. 103. For examples of the profession's pressures on legislatures and governors to establish sanitariums see *Transactions of the Medical Association of Georgia,* 51st ann. sess. (Atlanta, 1900), p. 53; ibid., 58th ann. sess. (Savannah, 1907), p. 53; T. E. Oertel, Remarks, ibid., 60th ann. sess. (Macon, 1909), pp. 42, 46; Editorial, *Calif. St. Jour. Med.* 3 (April 1905): 101; Editorial, *Jour. Mich. St. Med. Soc.* 4 (April 1905): 166; "Legislative Committee Report," *Texas St. Jour. Med.* 7 (June 1911): 49–50.

8. *Md. Med. Jour.* 51 (May 1908): 181; ibid. 51 (Dec. 1908): 544–45.

9. D. B. Hardenbergh, "County Hospital Law for Tuberculosis," *N.Y. St. Jour. Med.* 11 (April 1911): 180–81; W. E. McVey, "President's Address," *Jour. Kans. Med. Soc.* 4 (1 July 1904): 367, 372. For Connecticut's experiment with three hospitals in three different counties see Editorial, *Outlook* 92 (28 Aug. 1909): 962, and for Missouri's plan calling for district instead of county tuberculosis hospitals see "Report of the Committee on Public Policy and Legislation," *Jour. Mo. St. Med. Assn.* 8 (Aug. 1911): 78.

10. John B. Hawes II, "Educational Methods in the Anti-Tubercular Campaign," *Med. Com. Mass. Med. Soc.* 21, no. 4 (1910), p. 909; McVey, "President's Address," pp. 371–72. For a criticism of the federal government's greater concern for "our pigs" than "our children" see *N.Y. St. Jour. Med.* 7 (April 1907): 159.

11. Theodore Potter, "Report on Tuberculosis," *Transactions of the Indiana State Medical Association,* 55th ann. sess. (Richmond, 1904), p. 26; Theodore Potter, "Report on Tuberculosis," ibid., 56th ann. sess. (West Baden, 1905), pp. 466–67; Bonner, *Kansas Doctor,* p. 143. The movement to establish branches of the national association fighting tuberculosis seems to have gathered momentum late in the decade. The Michigan society, for example, established its branch in 1908, and the branch in the state of Washington held its first meeting that year. Aldred Scott Warthin, "The Organization of the State Anti-Tuberculosis Association," *Jour. Mich. St. Med. Soc.* 7 (March 1908): 119–20, and Editorial, *Northwest Med.* 6 (Feb. 1908): 68.

12. "Report of the Committee on the Prevention of Tuberculosis," *Pa. Med. Jour.* 14 (Oct. 1910): 57; *Transactions of the Medical Association of Georgia,* 61st ann. sess. (Athens, 1910), p. 32; Hawes, "Educational Methods in the Anti-Tuberculosis Campaign," p. 917.

13. Editorial, *Jour. Mich. St. Med. Soc.* 14 (June 1915): 324; "Report of the Committee on Tuberculosis," ibid. 15 (Sept. 1916): 454; Bonner, *Kansas Doctor,* pp. 143–46.

14. Letter, Frank Billings to editor, 24 Dec. 1906, *Ill. Med. Jour.* 11 (Jan. 1907): 59–60; Editorial, *Northwest Med.* 6 (June 1908): 235.

15. D. S. Lamb, "The Daily Medical Inspection of Schools," *N.Y. Med. Jour.* 74 (16 Nov. 1901): 923–25; S. W. Newmayer, "The Trained Nurse in the Public Schools as a Factor in the Education of Children," *Pa. Med. Jour.* 10 (Oct. 1906): 14; E. A. Montague, "Medical Inspection of Public Schools," *Northwest Med.,* n.s. 6 (June 1914): 174; S. D. Porter, Remarks, *New Orleans Med. Surg. Jour.* 67 (July 1914): 34; Martha Anderson, "Medical Inspection of Schools," *Ill. Med. Jour.* 3 (Feb. 1902): 420; E. B. Brown, "Medical Inspection of the Public Schools," *Wis. Med. Jour.* 14 (March 1916): 417. These writers disagree about the years when these cities started inspection, but the order presented here seems to be correct.

16. A. B. Montgomery, "Medical Inspection in Public Schools: Its Needs and Desirabilities," *Jour. Okla. Med. Assn.* 4 (Dec. 1911): 282; *Calif. St. Jour. Med.* 1 (Dec. 1903): 406; C. C. Wholey, "Education and School Inspection," *Pa. Med. Jour.* 9 (April 1906): 551.

17. Fletcher B. Dressler, Remarks, *Jour. Proc. Nat. Educ. Assn. U.S.,* 1912, p. 261; L. Rose Gantt, "Medical Inspection of Schools in Spartanburg, S.C.," *Jour. S.C. Med. Assn.* 7 (Sept. 1911): 329; Walter S. Cornell, Remarks, *Pa. Med. Jour.* 16 (Oct. 1912): 139.

18. Samuel G. Dixon, "Medical Inspection of School Children," *Pa. Med. Jour.* 15 (Sept. 1912): 940; *Ohio Med. Jour.* 4 (15 Feb. 1908): 108.

19. Edmund Moss, Remarks, *New Orleans Med. Surg. Jour.* 67 (July 1914): 32; Reed, "Medical Inspection of Schools," p. 275; Mary Gresham MacAdam, "The Benefits of Medical School Inspection," *N.Y. Med. Jour.* 71 (10 Feb. 1900): 181; *Transactions of the Medical Society of the State of New York* (Albany, 1903), p. 185.

20. S. D. Porter, Remarks, *New Orleans Med. Surg. Jour.* 67 (July 1914): 34–36; Cornell, Remarks, *Pa. Med. Jour.* 16 (Oct. 1912): 139.

21. Editorial, *Ohio St. Med. Jour.* 4 (15 July 1908): 427.

22. Reginald C. McGrane, *The Cincinnati Doctors' Forum* (Cincinnati: Academy of Medicine of Cincinnati, 1957), pp. 205, 207; "Report of the Councilor," *Jour. Mich. St. Med. Soc.* 8 [9] (Jan. 1910): 37, 38.

23. Editorial, *Calif. St. Jour. Med.* 5 (July 1907): 157.

24. *Calif. St. Jour. Med.* 9 (July 1911): 266; George H. Kress, "Medical Organization and Public Health Work, with a Special Application to the Milk Problem of California Cities," ibid. 5 (June 1907): 136–37; Kress, Remarks, ibid. 5 (Aug. 1907): 213. For a copy of the dairy score card used in the inspections see ibid. 5 (Sept. 1907): 243–44.

25. James G. Burrow, "The Prescription-Drug Policies of the American Medical Association in the Progressive Era," in John B. Blake, ed., *Safeguarding the Public* (Baltimore: The Johns Hopkins Press, 1970), p. 116; Editorial, *Texas St. Jour. Med.* 3 (May 1907): 3, 8–9; James G. Burrow, *AMA: Voice of American Medicine* (Baltimore: The Johns Hopkins Press, 1963), p. 63; R. W. Terhune, "Food Adulteration," *Transactions of the Indiana State Medical Association,* 1905, pp. 266–68; Editorials, *Calif. St. Jour. Med.* 4 (March 1906): 80; ibid. 4 (June 1906): 156; ibid. 5 (April

1907): 71; ibid. 5 (July 1907): 159. For a criticism of the advertising in the *Journal of the American Medical Association* see James Peter Warbasse, "Medical Journalism," *N.Y. St. Jour. Med.* 8 (Dec. 1908): 600. The struggle against nostrum advertising was won slowly. In 1911 the *Southern Medical Journal* (formerly *Gulf States Medical Journal*) announced that with the May issue it would "for the first time in the history of any medical journal in the South, present to its readers a medical periodical absolutely free from the taint of advertising any drug or medicine that is not favorably recognized by the U.S. Pharmacopoeia, the National Formulary, or New and Non-Official Remedies of the A.M.A. Council" (see Editorial, *Southern, Med. Jour.* 4 [May 1911]: 375).

26. For the profession's part in the passage and enforcement of this measure see Burrow, *AMA*, pp. 67–92, and for a comprehensive account of the first decade of its enforcement see James Harvey Young, *The Medical Messiahs* (Princeton: Princeton University Press, 1967), pp. 41–65.

27. T. B. Holloway, "Ophthalmia Neonatorum," *Pa. Med. Jour.* 17 (Dec. 1913): 187; Edward B. Heckel, "Ophthalmia Neonatorum and Its Relation to Blindness," *Pa. Med. Jour.* 16 (Jan. 1913): 280. For an attack by Abraham Jacobi and the profession generally on midwifery and for the methods employed to prevent ophthalmia neonatorum see *N.Y. St. Jour. Med.* 7 (April 1907): 164; F. Park Lewis, "Practical Legislation for the Prevention of Blindness and Ophthalmia Neonatorum," ibid., p. 134; and chapter 7 below.

28. Roswell Park, "The Work of the New York State Cancer Laboratory—Retrospective," *N.Y. St. Jour. Med.* 7 (May 1907): 186–87; ibid. 8 (March 1908): 145; Editorial, *Jour. Mich. St. Med. Soc.* 12 (March 1913): 169; letter, J. M. Wainswright to C. A. Thompson, *Okla. St. Med. Jour.* 7 (May 1915): 410–11; "Report of the Committee for the Control of Cancer," ibid. 8 (July 1915): 83.

29. "Report of the Committee on State Medicine and Hygiene," *Transactions of the Indiana State Medical Association,* 58th ann. sess. (Indianapolis, 1907), p. 455; Lewis Coleman Morris, "President's Address," *Transactions of the Medical Association of the State of Alabama* (Birmingham, 1912), p. 17.

30. *N.Y. St. Jour. Med.* 8 (Feb. 1908): 88; "Report of the Committee on the Pasteur Institute," *Trans Med. Assn. Ga.,* 1900, pp. 46, 47. For other examples of the profession's agitation for the creation and support of pathological laboratories see "Report of the Committee on Hygiene," *Transactions of the Medical Society of the State of New York* (Albany, 1904), p. 50; *N.Y. St. Jour. Med.* 11 (Feb. 1911): 92; A. P. Ohlmacher, "The Laboratory Movement in Ohio's State Hospitals," *Transactions of the Ohio State Medical Association,* 58th ann. sess. (Dayton, 1903), pp. 252, 254; "Report of the Board of Censors," *Transactions of the Medical Association of the State of Alabama* (Mobile, 1907), p. 87; *Trans. Ind. St. Med. Assn.,* 1905, pp. 470, 479.

31. "Report of the Committee on State Medicine and Hygiene," p. 437; A. B. Cooke, "Safeguarding Society from the Unfit," *Southern Med. Jour.* 3 (Dec. 1910): 17–20, quotation, p. 18; "Legislative Committee Report," *Texas St. Jour. Med.* 7 (June 1911): 51.

32. James E. Cassedy, "The Registration Area and American Vital Statistics: Development of a Health Insurance Resource, 1885–1915," *Bull. Hist. Med.* 39 (May-June 1965): 224, 225; George W. Webster, "Vital Statistics in Illinois," *Ill. Med. Jour.* 19 (Feb. 1911): 152; G. Farrar Patton, "Vital Statistics in Louisiana," *Transactions of the Louisiana State Medical Society,* 22d ann. sess. (New Orleans, 1901), p. 161. For criticism and defense of Alabama's method of collecting vital statistics see Lewis Coleman Morris, "President's Address," *Transactions of the Med-*

ical Association of the State of Alabama (Birmingham, 1912,) pp. 18–19; "Report of the Board of Censors," ibid., p. 67, and Charles A. Mohr, "A Plan for the Collection of Vital Statistics in Alabama," ibid. (Birmingham, 1909), pp. 535, 538.

33. Cassedy, "Registration Area," p. 223; Burrow, *AMA,* pp. 62–63; Editorial, *Ohio St. Med. Jour.* 5 (15 March 1909): 163.

34. Webster, "Vital Statistics in Illinois," pp. 152–53, 158; George William Williamson, "The Value of Vital Statistics to the Southern United States with Special Reference to Alabama," *Transactions of the Medical Association of the State of Alabama* (Mobile, 1913), p. 420; *JAMA* 74 (1 May 1920): 1241.

35. Burrow, *AMA,* pp. 94–95, 96n; Editorial, *Texas St. Jour. Med.* 4 (Nov. 1908): 168.

36. Burrow, *AMA,* pp. 98–100. For examples of the support that state society publications gave to the health department proposal see *Pa. Med. Jour.* 10 (June 1907): 698–701; Editorial, *Ill. Med. Jour.* 17 (Jan. 1910); 70–71; *Trans. Med. Assn. Ga.,* 1910, pp. 38–39; "The Revised Owen Bill and Its Opponents," *Okla. St. Med. Assn. Jour.* 4 (Dec. 1911): 306–7; Editorial, *Calif. St. Jour. Med.* 10 (Jan. 1912): 2–3; Editorial, *Jour. Mich. St. Med. Soc.* 11 (Sept. 1912): 597. For a regional publication's strong support see *Southern Med. Jour.* 3 (April 1910): 244–51, and Editorial, ibid. 3 (June 1910): 384–86.

37. Editorial, *Eclectic Med. Jour.* 71 (June 1911): 310.

38. Editorial, ibid. 70 (Sept. 1910): 470–71; Resolution, *Jour. AIH* 3 (Nov. 1910): 256; Editorial, ibid. 3 (Jan. 1911): 541; Editorial, *Calif. St. Jour. Med.* 10 (Jan. 1912): 2–3; Burrow, *AMA,* pp. 100–101; Manfred Waserman, "The Quest for a National Health Department in the Progressive Era," *Bull. Hist. Med.* 49 (Fall 1975): 371–76.

39. Allen F. Davis, *Spearheads for Reform: The Social Settlements and the Progressive Movement, 1890–1914* (New York: Oxford University Press, 1967), p. 132; Burrow, *AMA,* pp. 139n, 103–4; *JAMA* 59 (13 July 1912): 126.

CHAPTER SEVEN

1. The accusation most frequently raised against the AMA was that it had become a "medical trust"; for the protest of a prominent physician over the use of this epithet "all over the country," see J. A. Witherspoon's presidential address to the Tennessee State Medical Association appearing in *Jour. Tenn. St. Med. Assn.* 4 (May 1911): 3. In 1915 the federal Bureau of Corporations, which was being replaced by the Federal Trade Commission, stated that before 1890 the usual contract for reducing competition and gaining control of the market was "an agreement regarding production, or prices, or a pool." It added, "Such agreements, or pools took various forms, but frequently provided for some system of restricting output, or establishing a common selling agency" (Bureau of Corporations, United States Department of Agriculture, *Trust Laws and Unfair Competition* [Washington, D.C.: U.S. Government Printing Office, 1915], p. 5).

2. J. N. McCormack, "Medical Organization," *Transactions of the Tennessee State Medical Association,* 71st ann. sess. (Chattanooga, 1904), p. 62.

3. J. W. Gue, "Comments on Practice of Medicine," *Northwest Med.,* n.s. 5 (Nov. 1913): 301; Editorial, *Jour. Kans. Med. Soc. and Wichita Med. Jour.* 4 (1 Feb. 1904): 220; Editorial, *Ill. Med. Jour.* 14 (Aug. 1908): 229; John L. Irwin, "What Is to Become of the Medical Graduate [?]," *Jour. Mich. St. Med. Soc.* 3 (April 1904): 153–54; "Report of the Council on Medical Education," *Jour. Mo. St. Med Assn.* 7 (July 1910); 30.

4. Eliot Jones, *The Trust Problem in the United States* (New York: Macmillan

Co., 1929), pp. 199, 203, 229–30; Editorial, *Ill. Med. Jour.* 14 (Aug. 1908): 229; Editorial, *N.Y. St. Jour. Med.* 11 (Oct. 1911): 454.

5. Nathan B. Williams, comp., *Laws on Trusts and Monopolies Domestic and Foreign*, rev. ed. (Washington, D.C.: U.S. Government Printing Office, 1914), p. 119.

6. Jeremiah Whipple Jenks and Walter E. Clark, *The Trust Problem* (Garden City, N.Y.: Doubleday, Doran & Co., 1929), p. 213. These states were Maine, Michigan, North Carolina, and Tennessee (1889), and Kentucky, Mississippi, and South Dakota (1890).

7. Quotation in E. A. J. Johnson, *American Economic Thought in the Seventeenth Century* (New York: Russell & Russell, Inc., 1961), p. 130; Maurice Bear Gordon, *Aesculapius Comes to the Colonies* (Ventnor, N.J.: Ventnor Publishers, Inc., 1949), pp. 32–35. Richard B. Morris states that the Virginia law of 1639 was "constantly reenacted" (*Government and Labor in Early America* [New York: Octagon Books, Inc., 1965], p. 90).

8. A Louisiana law of 1890 exempted laborers in their efforts to raise wages. A revision of the California law in 1909 declared that labor was "not a commodity within the meaning of this act," and in 1913, Colorado made the same exclusion (Williams, comp., *Laws on Trusts and Monopolies*, pp. 64, 70, 141). In 1914 seven states, Delaware, Nevada, New Hampshire, Oregon, Pennsylvania, Rhode Island, and West Virginia, had neither constitutional provisions nor laws against trusts (Jenks and Clark, *Trust Problem*, p. 216).

9. J. N. McCormack, "A General Plan for a Schedule of Medical Fees," *Ill. Med. Jour.* 15 (Feb. 1909): 208; *Transactions of the Medical Association of the State of Alabama* (Mobile, 1910), p. 182. McCormack's fee schedule proposals originally appeared in *JAMA* 51 (28 Nov. 1908): 1882–83.

10. "Secretary's Report," *Texas St. Jour. Med.* 3 (June 1907): 62–64; Editorial, ibid. 2 (Aug. 1906): 102; "Course in Medical Economics," *JAMA* 48 (19 June 1907): 246–47.

11. *Jour. Kans. Med. Soc.* 6 (1 July 1906): 299.

12. Ibid. 4 (1 Jan. 1904): 176. For similar instructions that Joseph N. McCormack gave the Texas Medical Association see *Texas St. Jour. Med.* 1 (Dec. 1905): 219.

13. Collaboration with irregular physicians became easier after 1903 when the AMA replaced its medical code with the "Principles of Medical Ethics" allowing state societies to permit their members to engage in medical consultation with members of some irregular groups and to grant membership to physicians adhering to no exclusive system. See James G. Burrow, *AMA: Voice of American Medicine* (Baltimore: The Johns Hopkins Press, 1963), p. 33n, and Donold E. Konold, *A History of American Medical Ethics, 1847–1912* (Madison: The State Historical Society of Wisconsin, 1962), pp. 68–69.

14. *Ill. Med. Jour.* 11 (May 1907): 551. On the matter of publicizing fee schedules an eastern journal admonished, "A fee bill is an instrument which should be retained in our own hands as a guide in fixing charges; it should never, under any circumstances, be made public" (Editorial, *N.Y. St. Jour. Med.* 12 [June 1912]: 277).

15. *N.Y. Med. Jour.* 86 (24 Aug. 1907): 365.

16. Editorial, *Ill. Med. Jour.* 11 (Jan. 1907): 55; *Pa. Med. Jour.* 10 (Oct. 1906): 59–60.

17. See, for example, p. 26 above.

18. McCormack, "General Plan," pp. 205–8.

19. Ibid. pp. 205–6.

20. "Articles of Agreement," *Ky. Med. Jour.* 6 (Feb. 1908): 103–4. Appendix VI gives this agreement in full. For a case in which physicians were fined $25 for calling on blacklisted people see *JAMA* 39 (1 Nov. 1902): 1120, which cites the plan adopted by the Moline City Hospital in Illinois.

21. G. Frank Lydston, "Medicine as a Business Proposition," *Colo. Med. Jour. and Western Gaz.* 6 (June 1900): 250; Linsly R. Williams, "The Value of the Social Worker and the Visiting Nurse to the Dispensary Patient," *N.Y. Med. Jour.* 87 (25 Jan. 1908): 143; "Report on the Investigation of One Thousand Dispensary Patients," *N.Y. St. Jour. Med.* 13 (Jan. 1913): 48; quotation, Howard D. King, "Hospital Abuse in New Orleans," *New Orleans Med. Surg. Jour.* 66 (Jan. 1914): 555.

22. Edith P. de Veaux, "Free Dispensaries and Their Abuse," *Northwest Med.* 2 (April 1904): 151.

23. *Ill. Med. Jour.* 19 (Feb. 1911): 257; *Jour. Mich. St. Med. Soc.* 4 (Feb. 1905): 78, quotation, p. 79. For other objections to the discount policies of university hospitals see Joseph Price, "The Irregular Regular in Public and Hospital Practice," *Pa. Med. Jour.* 10 (Nov. 1906): 133; John Sunwall, "The University Health Fee," *Jour. Kans. Med. Soc.* 15 (Oct. 1915): 314–19.

24. Anne Moore, "Report of Committee on Dispensary Abuse, 1912," *N.Y. St. Jour. Med.* 13 (Jan. 1913), quotation, p. 50, see also pp. 48–50.

25. Charles S. Stockton, "The Future of Medicine," *Ill. Med. Jour.* 18 (July 1910): 1; ibid. 19 (Feb. 1911): 257.

26. Moore, "Report on Dispensary Abuse," pp. 52–53; Florence Larrabee Lattimore, "The Medical Charities of Manhattan and the Bronx," *N.Y. St. Jour. Med.* 7 (Feb. 1907): 49; *JAMA* 37 (5 Oct. 1901): 916.

27. Lloyd A. Clary, "A Few Remarks on Proprietary Medicines and the Relation of Doctor and Patient," *Jour. Kans. Med. Soc.* 7 (1 Nov. 1907): 1124–25; Julius H. Comroe, "Prescribing versus Dispensing," *Pa. Med. Jour.* 12 (Oct. 1908): 24–31.

28. J. N. McCormack, "What Should Be the Relations of Pharmacists and Physicians [?]," *Texas St. Jour. Med.* 3 (Oct. 1907): 167–68.

29. Comroe, "Prescribing," pp. 24–25; Clary, "Remarks on Proprietary Medicines," p. 1125; Editorial, *Jour. Mo. St. Med. Assn.* 5 (Sept. 1908): 176.

30. Clary, "Remarks on Proprietary Medicines," p. 1124; Comroe, "Prescribing," p. 26.

31. Charles E. Seivers, "What Are We Going to Do about It [?]," *Jour. Kans. Med. Soc.* 13 (Oct. 1913): 411; Comroe, "Prescribing," p. 31.

32. McCormack, "What Should Be the Relations," p. 167. McCormack had criticized the pharmaceutical industry in his report to the annual session of the House of Delegates in 1907. He was invited to speak to the American Pharmaceutical Association explaining his criticism. This quotation comes from the original criticism which he repeated at this meeting (see "Report of the Committee on Organization," *JAMA* 48 [15 June 1907]: 2044).

33. McCormack, "What Should Be the Relations," p. 167.

34. Comroe, "Prescribing," p. 27.

35. *Texas St. Jour. Med.* 3 (Dec. 1907): 218. This account is reprinted from an unidentified issue of *JAMA*.

36. For a detailed account of the AMA's struggle with the patent-medicine forces in this era see Burrow, *AMA*, pp. 67–131, or for a summary of the early part of the struggle see Frank Billings, "The Nostrum Evil," *Pa. Med. Jour.* 9 (Dec. 1905): 211–12.

37. Maurice J. Lewi, "What Shall Be Done with the Professional Midwife?" *Transactions of the Medical Society of the State of New York* (Albany, 1902), pp.

282–83; Francis E. Kobrin, "The American Midwife Controversy: A Crisis of Professionalization," *Bull. Hist. Med.* 40 (July–Aug. 1966): 350, 358.

38. *N.Y. Med. Jour.* 71 (21 April 1900): 622; Resolution, *Transactions of the Louisiana State Medical Association,* 22d ann. sess. (New Orleans, 1901), pp. 24, 25.

39. Lewi, "The Professional Midwife," pp. 362–63.

40. Kobrin, "American Midwife Controversy," pp. 362–63.

CHAPTER EIGHT

1. Frederick D. Mott and Milton Roemer, *Rural Health and Medical Care* (New York: McGraw-Hill Book Co., 1948), pp. 437–38; George Rosen, *Fees and Fee Schedules in Nineteenth Century America,* in *Supplement to Bull. Hist Med.,* No. 6, Henry E. Sigerist, ed. (Baltimore: The Johns Hopkins Press, 1946), p. 25; Donald E. Konold, *A History of American Medical Ethics, 1847–1912* (Madison: The State Historical Society of Wisconsin, 1962), pp. 57–58.

2. "Report of the Committee on Contract Practice," *Jour. Mich. St. Med. Soc.* 6 (April 1906): 132–35; "Minority Report of Committee on Contract Practice," *Calif. St. Jour. Med.* 9 (Dec. 1911): 507; Charles M. Emmons, "Medical Ethics and Commercialism," *Southern Med. Jour.* 2 (July 1909); 853; Albert T. Lytle, "Contract Medical Practice—An Economic Study," *N.Y. St. Jour. Med.* 15 (March 1915): 104.

3. "Report of the Committee on Contract Practice," *Jour. Mich. St. Med. Soc.* 6 (July 1907): 377–78; George Archibald Hogan, Article, *Transactions of the Medical Association of the State of Alabama* (State Board of Health) (Montgomery, 1905), p. 452; "Forty-second Annual Report of the Boards of Censors," ibid. (Birmingham, 1915), pp. 129–30; Horace M. Alleman, "Lodge Practice," *Pa. Med. Jour.* 15 (Dec. 1911): 223; Editorial, *N.Y. Med. Jour.* 92 (Nov. 1910): 810; "Report of the Judicial Council," *JAMA* 60 (21 June 1913): 1997; "Special Report on Health Insurance," *Texas St. Jour. Med.* 12 (June 1916): 88.

4. "Report of the Committee on Contract Practice," *Jour. Mich. St. Med. Soc.* 6 (July 1907): 378–79.

5. "Report of the Committee on Contract Work of the Medical Society of the County of Erie," *N.Y. St. Jour. Med.* 11 (Aug. 1911): 394–95; "Report of the Committee on Dispensary Abuse, 1912," ibid., 13 (Jan. 1913): 54; Editorial comment from unidentified issue of the *Cleveland Medical Journal,* in *Md. Med. Jour.* 54 (Feb. 1911): c; George E. Holtzapple, "Lodge Practice," *Pa. Med. Jour.* 11 (April 1908): 533–35. In May 1916, John V. Woodruff, a physician of Buffalo, said that 240,000 of the population of that city had access to the services of lodge physicians ("Contract Practice," *N.Y. St. Jour. Med.* 16 [Oct. 1916]: 508).

6. Undated letter, R. Y. Ferguson to the Secretary, *Jour. Mich. St. Med. Soc.* 7 (May 1908): 267; "Report of the Committee on Contract Practice," ibid. 6 (July 1907): 378, 380; Charles J. Whalen, "The Abuse of Medical Charities in Chicago," *Ill. Med. Jour.* 15 (Jan. 1909): 10; *Report of the Health Insurance Commission of the State of Illinois* (Springfield, 1 May 1919), p. 524; W. W. Anderson, Remarks, *Ky. Med. Jour.* 6 (Oct. 1908): 594.

7. Editorial, *Northwest Med.* 4 (April 1906): 133.

8. *Calif. St. Jour. Med.* 4 (Feb. 1906): 37; Rexwald Brown, "Evils of the Lodge Practice System." ibid. 6 (April 1908): 127.

9. Whalen, "Abuse of Charities," p. 5; Editorial, *Northwest Med.* 5 (Jan. 1907): 33; "Report of the Committee on Contract and Lodge Practice," *Calif. St. Jour. Med.* 9 (June 1911): 233–34. The American Hospital Association referred to here appears to be no more than a small promotional organization with an impressive name.

10. "Minority Report of the Committee on Contract Practice," p. 507; Emmons,

"Medical Ethics," p. 851. For the experience of the Michigan State Medical Society with contracts providing medical care to the poor see "Report of the Committee on Contract Practice," p. 379–80.

11. Holtzapple, "Lodge Practice," pp. 530–33.

12. "Report of the Committee on Contract Practice," p. 378; letter, R. Y. Ferguson to the Secretary, *Jour. Mich. St. Med. Soc.* 7 (May 1908): 267; T. M. Johnson, "The Business Side of the Profession of Medicine," *Ohio St. Med. Jour.* 1 (15 June 1906): 583; Whalen, "Abuse of Charities," p. 11.

13. "Report of the Committee on Ethics of the San Francisco Medical Society," *Calif. St. Jour. Med.* 2 (May 1904): 166; ibid. 2 (Feb. 1906): 45; Editorial, *Northwest Med.* 5 (Jan. 1907): 33.

14. Whalen, "Abuse of Charities," p. 11; "Report of the Judicial Council," *JAMA* 60 (21 June 1913): 1997; quotation, Editorial, *Jour. Mich. St. Med. Soc.* 8 (Sept. 1909): 417.

15. "Report of the Board of Censors," *Transactions of the Medical Association of the State of Alabama* (Birmingham, 1890), pp. 75–79; "Twenty-Seventh Annual Report of the Board of Censors," ibid. (Montgomery, 1900), pp. 88–89.

16. Provision of medical care for tenants presented a problem that some local societies in Texas discussed with farm organizations early in the twentieth century. Few societies over the nation appear to have recognized the problem. For the situation in Texas see J. N. McCormack, "The Great Work Being Done in Texas," *Texas St. Jour. Med.* 2 (May 1906): 30.

17. Sterling D. Shimer, "Thoughts, Here and There," *Pa. Med. Jour.* 11 (July 1908): 809; Editorial, *Ohio St. Med. Jour.* 1 (15 Feb. 1906): 386. The Committee on Railroad Contract Practice of the Texas state association took a different view on the issue of railroad remuneration from that presented here. In 1909 it reported that in many cases the free pass was adequate compensation. It also stated that surgeons often received from the railroads 50 to 75 percent of their normal charges, but that with guaranteed pay the amount received was about equal to or even above that secured for comparable service in regular practice (see "Report of the Committee on Railroad Contract Practice," *Texas St. Jour. Med.* 5 [June 1909]: 70).

18. For examples of criticisms by journals and societies of these practices see "Contract Practice," *JAMA* 57 (8 July 1911): 145; John Clark LeGrand, "President's Address," *Transactions of the Medical Association of the State of Alabama* (Montgomery, 1900), p. 27; "Thirty-fourth Annual Report of the Board of Censors," ibid. (Mobile, 1907), p. 86; E. T. Camp, "Some Problems Confronting the Medical Profession," ibid. (Birmingham, 1913), p. 441.

19. "Twenty-seventh Annual Report," *Trans. Med. Assn. St. Ala.*, 1900, p. 89; Camp, "Problems Confronting the Profession," p. 435.

20. Whalen, "Abuse of Charities," p. 8; quotation, *Calif. St. Jour. Med.* 4 (Feb. 1906): 45.

21. "Report of the Committee on Contract and Lodge Practice," p. 234.

22. "Medical Economics," *JAMA* 51 (1 Aug. 1908): 425.

23. Alleman, "Lodge Practice," p. 223; Brown, "Evils of Lodge Practice," p. 126.

24. "Report of the Committee on Contract and Lodge Practice," p. 234.

25. See, for instance, the bylaws adopted by the Medico-Legal Society of Philadelphia in 1905 and the resolution of the King County Medical Association in Washington in 1906 (*Pa. Med. Jour.* 9 [Nov. 1905]: 129, and Editorial, *Northwest Med.* 4 [April 1906]: 134).

26. *Calif. St. Jour. Med.* 10 (June 1912): 229, 232.

27. "Contract Practice," *JAMA* 57 (8 July 1911): 145–46.

28. "Report of the Judicial Council," *JAMA* 60 (21 June 1913): 1997, quotation, p. 1998. Donald E. Konold states that when the AMA revised its "Principles of Medical Ethics" in 1912 it "outlawed contract practice below standard rates" that physicians charged. The Judicial Council drafted a revision of the ethics in 1912, and Article VI, Section 3, stated, "It is not advisable for a county medical society to establish a fee bill; when, however, as is frequently the case, the physicians in a town or community agree upon the minimum fee to be accepted from their patients as a return for their services, honorable conduct demands adherence to this agreement." The Reference Committee on Amendments to Constitution and By-Laws would not accept this provision, and the revised document which the House of Delegates accepted at this meeting omitted this section (Konold, *History of Medical Ethics*, p. 71; *Proceedings of the House of Delegates of the American Medical Association*, 63rd ann. sess. [Atlantic City, 1912], pp. 4, 15, 47).

29. *JAMA* 60 (28 June 1913): 2084–85; quotation, "Report of the Judicial Council," *JAMA* 60 (21 June 1913): 1998.

30. J. T. Richardson, *The Origin and Development of Group Hospitalization in the United States, 1890–1940*, University of Missouri Studies, vol. 20, no. 3 (Columbia: University of Missouri Press, 1945), p. 14. For an account of the promotional scheme of a hospital association see Editorial, *Calif. St. Jour. Med.* 11 (Oct. 1913): 389.

31. Resolution, *Calif. St. Jour. Med.* 10 (June 1912): 229.

32. Ibid.

33. E. Eliot Harris, "A Plea for the Betterment of the Economic Condition of Medicine," *N.Y. St. Jour. Med.* 13 (Feb. 1913): 78, 80–81; Editorial, *Jour. Mich. St. Med. Soc.* 12 (Jan. 1913): 41. For McCormack's ideas see p. 21 above.

34. "Committee to Investigate Contract Work of the Medical Society of the County of Erie," *N.Y. St. Jour. Med.* 11 (Aug. 1911): 395, 394.

35. Ibid., pp. 395, 396.

36. Zierath, "Contract Practice," *Wis. Med. Jour.* 6 (Aug. 1907): 161.

37. "Report of the Committee to Define Contract Practice," *Pa. Med. Jour.* 15 (Feb. 1912): 415. See also note 25 above.

38. Resolution, *Jour. Mich. St. Med. Soc.* 6 (June 1907): 303; Editorial, ibid. 6 (July 1907): 365; A. B. Hirsh, Remarks, *Pa. Med. Jour.* 12 (Dec. 1908): 234; Editorial, *Calif. St. Jour. Med.* 11 (Feb. 1913): 41.

CHAPTER NINE

1. Frederick L. Van Sickle, "The Relation of the Medical Profession to the Workmen's Compensation Acts of the United States," *Pa. Med. Jour.* 17 (April 1914): 877; I. M. Rubinow, *Social Insurance* (New York: Henry Holt and Co., 1913), pp. 156, 174. New York's workmen's compensation law of 1910 that was declared unconstitutional the next year ushered in, according to Rubinow, "the modern era of compensation acts in American states" (ibid., p. 171). For very limited compensation laws passed in Maryland in 1902, and in Montana in 1909, which were declared unconstitutional, and for a federal compensation act in 1908 with limited application see ibid., pp. 157, 170–71, 159.

2. Herman Miles Somers and Anne Ramsay Somers, *Workmen's Compensation: Prevention, Insurance and Rehabilitation of Occupational Diseases* (New York: John Wiley & Sons, 1954), p. 23; W. H. Allport, "Employers' Liability Insurance," *Ill. Med. Jour.* 17 (May 1910): 712–13.

3. Roy Lubove, *The Struggle for Social Security, 1900–1935* (Cambridge: Harvard University Press, 1968), pp. 50–51. For an elaborate treatment of American

modifications of common law applicable to industrial injuries see Crystal Eastman, *Work-Accidents and the Law* (New York: Charities Publication Committee, 1910), pp. 169–89.

4. Eastman, *Work-Accidents and the Law*, p. 121; Arthur Larson, "Compensation Reform in the United States," in Earl F. Cheit and Margaret S. Gordon, eds., *Occupational Disability and Public Policy* (New York: John Wiley & Sons, 1963), p. 17.

5. Francis D. Donoghue, "Medical Services and Medical and Hospital Fees under Workmen's Compensation," U.S. Department of Labor, Bureau of Labor Statistics, *Proceedings of the Conference on Social Insurance, 1916, Bulletin of the United States Bureau of Labor Statistics Whole Number 212* (Washington, D.C.: U.S. Government Printing Office, 1917), p. 310; Editorial, *Wis. Med. Jour.* 14 (Jan. 1916): 361. Actually by 1 January 1915 more than half of the states had enacted compensation statutes; by May 1916 the number had reached thirty-three and remained at that number in February 1917. I. M. Rubinow, "Standards of Health Insurance," reprint from the *Journal of Political Economy* 23 (March, April, and May 1915): 221; John B. McAlister, "How the Workmen's Compensation Act May Be Made Satisfactory to the Profession," *Pa. Med. Jour.* 19 (July 1916): 736; Frank B. Walker, "Social Insurance," *Jour. Mich. St. Med. Soc.* 16 (May 1917): 200.

6. Editorial, *Calif. St. Jour. Med.* 12 (Jan. 1914): 4; Editorial, ibid. 12 (Feb. 1914): 48; ibid. 12 (May 1914): 196a; Burton R. Corbus, "Social Legislation and the Doctor," *Jour. Mich. St. Med. Soc.* 12 (March 1913): 152–53.

7. "Report of the Committee on Industrial Accident Insurance", *Calif. St. Jour. Med.* 15 (July 1917): 198–99. For examples of reports showing that the free-choice principle had been undermined see Charles H. Crounhart, Paper, *Wis. Med. Jour.* 14 (Dec. 1915): 272, and William A. Schnader, "The Pennsylvania Workmen's Compensation Legislation; How It Affects the Physician, the Surgeon and the Hospital," *Pa. Med. Jour.* 19 (March 1916): 401.

8. Van Sickle, "Medical Profession," p. 884; W. F. Zierath, "The Ninety Day Clause in the Workmen's Compensation Act," *Wis. Med. Jour.* 13 (May 1915): 483–84; Editorial, ibid. 13 (June 1914): 25; Editorial, *Northwest Med.*, n.s. 4 (May 1912): 156; *Okla. St. Med. Jour.* 8 (Dec. 1915): 248. In September 1914, H. Eugene Allen, a Seattle physician, reported that after passage of the compensation law, suits in Washington had increased 700 percent and that all of the reliable companies had ceased to write physicians' liability insurance in the state. "They gave as their reason that they cannot buck the conditions brought on by the Compensation Act in this state even at increased premiums" ("State Industrial Insurance in Washington," *Northwest Med.*, n.s. 7 [Jan. 1915]: 24). One medical editor cited a personal injury accident in which the victim received letters from forty lawyers wishing to institute legal proceedings (Editorial, *Wis. Med. Jour.* 13 [June 1914]: 25).

9. Crounhart, Paper, *Wis. Med. Jour.* 14 (Dec. 1915): 272.

10. Editorial, *Calif. St. Jour. Med.* 12 (Jan. 1914): 4; Resolution adopted by the councilors of the Los Angeles County Medical Society, ibid. 3 (March 1914): 125; *Editorial, Northwest Med.*, n.s. 4 (May 1912): 157.

11. Editorial, *Jour. Mich. St. Med. Soc.* 13 (June 1914): 403. Ohio presented an exceptional case where physicians appeared to have been better paid and raised fewer complaints. The Ohio Industrial Commission collected fixed premiums and made awards (C. D. Selby, A. W. Bruckley, and J. W. Means, "The Ohio Workmen's Compensation Act: Report of Committee from the Surgical Section," *Ohio St. Jour. Med.* 10 [July 1914]: 415, but see also ibid., p. 420).

12. Resolution of Los Angeles County Society, p. 125; Editorial, ibid. 13 (June 1914): 403; "Preliminary Report of the Workmen's Compensation Commission," *N.Y. St. Jour. Med.* 14 (Aug. 1914): 425.

13. McAlister, "Workmen's Compensation Act," p. 738; Van Sickle, "Medical Profession," p. 885; quotation, Editorial, *Jour. Mich. St. Med. Soc.* 13 (June 1914): 403. The Michigan society had no schedule for workmen's compensation. Its House of Delegates twice had rejected schedules drawn up by committees appointed for that purpose (Editorial, *Jour. Mich. St. Med. Soc.* 15 [Sept. 1916]: 460). In Massachusetts a real crisis developed over the compensation schedule requiring intervention by the governor who appointed a commission to fix the schedule. See letter, Bert Nottingham to F. C. Warnshius, 25 Sept. 1913, *Jour. Mich. St. Med. Soc.* 12 (Nov. 1913): 621.

14. Resolution, *Calif. St. Jour. Med.* 12 (March 1914): 125; H. M. Dunham, "Does the Workmen's Compensation Law Change the Old Time Relation between the Physician and His Patient?" *Jour. Mich. St. Med. Soc.* 13 (Jan. 1914): 58; quotation, Allen, "Insurance in Washington," p. 24. For treatment of the concept of "privileged communications," see Elmer D. Brothers, *Medical Jurisprudence,* 2d ed. (St. Louis: C. V. Mosley Co., 1925), pp. 46–52.

15. For the emphasis that the AALL placed on compulsory health insurance as the next most urgent need in social legislation see John B. Andrews to Frederic W. Loughram, 18 Jan. 1916, American Association for Labor Legislation, John B. Andrews Papers, Record Group A-1, Correspondence, 1916, Box 14, Library of the New York State School of Industrial and Labor Relations, Cornell University, Ithaca, N.Y.; "Health Insurance: Next Great Step in Social Legislation," Press Release, 25 Sept. 1916, announcing address of John B. Andrews before the Minnesota Conference on Charities and Correction, Andrews Papers, RG A-1, Correspondence, 1916, Box 15; Isaac Max Rubinow to A. M. Simons, 14 July 1932, p. 2, Isaac Max Rubinow Collection, A-3, Correspondence SA-TZ, Box 8, Library of the New York State School of Industrial and Labor Relations, Cornell University; J. R. Commons, "Health Insurance," *Wis. Med. Jour.* 18 (Nov. 1918): 220. Materials from the files of the American Association for Labor Legislation cited above will be referred to hereafter as the Andrews and Rubinow Papers.

16. *Amer. Labor. Leg. Rev.* 4 (Dec. 1914): 511; Editorial, ibid. 2 (Feb. 1912): 164–65; *Who's Who in America,* vol. 9 (1916–17), p. 57. From the beginning men of distinction and scholarship filled important positions in the AALL. Richard T. Ely, a prominent social scientist, served as its first president. The first issue of its official organ listed Henry R. Seager of Columbia University as president, and Louis D. Brandeis, Samuel Gompers, and Woodrow Wilson as among the vice presidents. See inside front cover, *Amer. Labor. Leg. Rev.* 1 (Jan. 1911); and Editorial, ibid. 2 (Feb. 1912): 512, for Ely's election.

17. John B. Andrews, "Progress toward Health Insurance," *Proceedings of the National Conference on Social Work,* 34th ann. sess. (Pittsburgh, 1917), p. 535; "Secretary's Report," *Amer. Labor Leg. Rev.* 6 (March 1916): 104; ibid. 4 (Dec. 1914): 578; Rubinow, *Social Insurance,* pp. 169–70; I. M. Rubinow, "Social Insurance," *Amer. Labor Leg. Rev.* 3 (June 1913): 163.

18. Harold U. Faulkner, *The Decline of Laissez Faire, 1897–1914,* Economic History of the United States, vol. 7, ed. Henry David et al. (New York: Holt, Rinehart and Winston, 1951), pp. 251–53. In 1916 the AALL showed that in Washington, D.C., the public spent annually about $500,000 on health insurance collected by agents in amounts varying from ten to twenty-five cents, but that only about

$200,000 reached the insured annually in benefits. The high cost of securing business and making collections took much of the balance ("Brief for Health Insurance," *Amer. Labor Leg. Rev.* 6 [June 1916]: 199).

19. In 1912, Theodore Roosevelt's Progressive party got 4,119,507 votes and the Socialist party 901,873; thus, of the four leading parties, these two got 29 percent of the votes cast. The Progressive platform called for "the protection of home life against the hazards of sickness, irregular employment and old age through the adoption of a system of social insurance adapted to American use." The Socialist platform favored "a general system of insurance by the states of all of its members against unemployment and invalidism." For platforms see Kirk H. Porter and Donald Bruce Johnson, *National Party Platforms, 1840–1960*, 2d ed. (Urbana: University of Illinois Press, 1961), pp. 177, 190, and for election results, Arthur S. Link, *Wilson: The Road to the White House* (Princeton: Princeton University Press, 1947), pp. 524–25.

20. B. S. Warren and Edgar Sydenstricker, "Health Insurance: Its Relation to the Public Health," U.S. Treasury Department, *United States Public Health Bulletin No. 76, March 1916* (Washington, D.C.: U.S. Government Printing Office, 1916), p. 65; Robert T. Legge, "Students' Health Insurance at the University of California," Department of Labor, *Proceedings of the Conference on Social Insurance*, 1916, pp. 505–11.

21. The AALL began collecting material on health insurance for the model bill in 1912 (*New York Times Magazine*, 30 Jan. 1916, p. 8).

22. The AALL was far more than a small organization of educators though the leadership lay largely with this class. In 1914 it had a paid membership of 3,058 with receipts totaling nearly $28,000 (Statement prepared 7 Jan. 1916, Andrews Papers, RG A-1, Corres., 1916, Box 14).

23. Quotation in Robert A. Allen, "State Insurance against Sickness," *JAMA* 63 (11 July 1914): 186, and James P. Warbasse, "What is the Matter with the Medical Profession?" *Long Island Med. Jour.* 6 (July 1912): 275; "Twenty-eighth Report of the Board of Censors," *Transactions of the Medical Association of the State of Alabama* (Selma, 1901), p. 108; *N.Y. St. Jour. Med.* 11 (Jan. 1911): 42; E. Eliot Harris, "A Plan for the Betterment of the Economic Conditions of Medicine," ibid. 13 (Feb. 1913): 78–81. Although these organizations had not been formed to advance compulsory health insurance, their establishment showed growing concern for a wide range of economic and social issues affecting medicine.

24. C. E. Mattison, "President's Address," *Calif. St. Jour. Med.* 12 (June 1914): 224–25. Mattison was not alone in foreseeing an era of compulsory health insurance. In May 1914 the board of directors of the National Association of Manufacturers requested Fred C. Schwedtman to gather materials on health insurance and to report on his findings. In his report of 1 July he said: "*I give it as my opinion that Sickness Insurance of some kind, with compulsory contributions on the part of employers, will be enacted into law by many States of the Union within the next five years and that now is the time to go into this subject and carry on an educational campaign such as we have been carrying on in connection with Workmen's Compensation Insurance and Accident Prevention*" (*To the President and the Board of Directors, National Association of Manufacturers*, 1 July 1914, pamphlet, Andrews Papers, RG A-1, Health Insurance, Box 70).

25. "Preliminary Standards for Sickness Insurance Recommended by the Committee on Social Insurance," *Amer. Labor Leg. Rev.* 4 (Dec. 1914): 595; "Secretary's Report," ibid. 6 (March 1916): 104; John R. Commons, "Social Insurance and the Medical Profession," *Wis. Med. Jour.* 13 (Jan. 1915): 301–6; W. F. Zierath,

"The Socialization of Medicine," ibid., pp. 306–11; C. S. Sheldon, "President's Address," ibid. 13 (Oct. 1914): 180; I. M. Rubinow, "Social Insurance and the Medical Profession," *JAMA* 64 (30 Jan. 1915): 381–86. A report of Rubinow's address appears in Rubinow Papers, RG A-3, Box 10.

26. Editorial, *Calif. St. Jour. Med.* 13 (June 1915): 214; Editorial, *JAMA* 67 (2 Dec. 1916): 1677.

27. Philip Mills Jones to Andrews, 15 Dec. 1915, Andrews Papers, RG A-1, 1915, Box 13; Andrews to T. W. Grayson, 7 Jan. 1915, Andrews Papers, RG A-1, Corres., 1916, Box 14; *Amer. Labor Leg. Rev.* 6 (March 1916): 104–5. In an undated three-page draft in the Rubinow Papers, Rubinow summarizes his work including his connection with the AMA's Social Insurance Committee (see RG A-3, Corres., PI-RZ, Box 7).

28. Warren and Sydenstricker, "Health Insurance," pp. 76, 206–7. For a brief account of the work of this commission and of the eleven volumes of its findings published in 1916 see Allen F. Davis, *Spearheads for Reform: The Social Settlements and the Progressive Movement, 1890–1914* (New York: Oxford University Press, 1968), pp. 208–17.

29. OSH [Olga S. Halsey] to Philip Mills Jones, 5 Jan. 1916, Andrews Papers, RG A-1, Corres., 1916, Box 14; *Report of the Insurance Commission of the State of Illinois, May 1, 1919*, p. 5. It was probably in 1915 when the Progressive National Service published an impressive sixty-page pamphlet entitled *Sickness Insurance*. The name of the author is not given, but a copy in the Andrews Papers is inscribed on the front by J. P. Chamberlain (see RG A-1, Health Insurance, Box 70). For additional information on the Progressive National Service see Davis, *Spearheads for Reform*, pp. 206–8, 213–16, though he mistakenly refers to it as the "National Progressive Service."

30. Lambert's secretary (Gertrude Cuthill) to Olga S. Halsey, 6 Jan. 1916; OSH to Craig, 7 Jan. 1916; Andrews to Fisher, 18 Jan. 1916; Andrews to Lambert, 19 Jan. 1916, Andrews Papers, RG A-1, Corres., 1916, Box 14. By the end of January the AALL had circulated thirteen thousand copies of the health insurance bill (John B. Andrews, "Health Insurance," *Proceedings of the National Association for the Study and Prevention of Tuberculosis* [Washington, D.C., 1916], p. 6, reprint in Andrews Papers, RG A-1, Papers of the Society, Box 68).

31. For the model bill as it appeared in June 1916 see Committee on Social Insurance of AALL, "Health Insurance: Tentative Draft of an Act," *Amer. Labor Leg. Rev.* 6 (June 1916): 238–68, and for a summary see Alexander Lambert, "Provisions for Medical Care under Health Insurance," *Texas St. Jour. Med.* 12 (Oct. 1916): 249–51. Lambert's article is a reprint from *The Modern Hospital*, Aug. 1916.

32. Lambert, "Provisions for Medical Care," pp. 250–51; OSH to Julia Lathrop, 3 Feb. 1916, Andrews Papers, RG A-1, Corres., 1916, Box 14.

33. *N.E. Med. Gaz.* 51 (April 1916): 219–20, 288–90; A. C. Burnham, "A Plan for the Care of the Insured under the Proposed Health Insurance Law," reprint from *Med. Record*, 22 April 1916, Andrews Papers, RG A-1, Health Insurance, Box 70; OSH to T. D. Patterson, 13 April 1916, Andrews Papers, RG A-1, Corres., 1916, Box 14; I. M. Rubinow, "Health Insurance in Relation to the Public Dispensary," reprint, Andrews Papers, RG A-1, Box 70.

34. Andrews to Blumer, 3 May 1916, Blumer to Andrews, 23 May 1916, Blumer File, Health Insurance, 1915–19, Yale Medical Historical Library, New Haven, Conn.; *Pa. Med. Jour.* 19 (July 1916): 756–58; *Proceedings of the Connecticut State Medical Society* (Bridgeport, 1916), pp. 87–89; B. S. Warren to Andrews, 25 May 1916, Andrews Papers, RG A-1, Corres., 1916, Box 14; United States Public

Health Service, *Health Insurance: Report of Standing Committee Adopted by the Conference on State and Territorial Health Authorities with the United States Public Health Service*, Washington, D.C., 13 May 1916 (Washington, D.C.: U.S. Government Printing Office, 1916), pp. 1–8.

35. For the address see *Health Insurance*, quotation, p. 9.

36. Andrews, form letter, 16 May, 1916, Andrews Papers, RG A-1, Corres., 1916, Box 14.

37. I. M. Rubinow, "The Relation between Private and Social Insurance," reprint from *Proceedings of the Casualty, Actuarial and Statistical Society of America*, vol. 2, pt. 3, no. 6, p. 342, Andrews Papers, RG A-1, Health Insurance, Box 70.

38. I. M. Rubinow, "Health Insurance in Its Relation to Public Health," reprint from *JAMA* 67 (16 Sept. 1916): 1011–15, Rubinow Papers, RG A-3, Box 10.

39. Editorial, *Jour. Mich. St. Med. Soc.* 15 (July 1916): 350–56; Editorial, ibid. 15 (Aug. 1916): 398–402; "Report of the Interim Committee on Health Insurance," *Wis. Med. Jour.* 15 (Dec. 1916): 226; "Report of the Committee on Social Insurance," ibid. 16 (Jan. 1918): 281; H. E. Dearholt, Remarks, ibid. 17 (Nov. 1918): 232.

40. Jones to Andrews, 22 and 26 April 1916, Andrews Papers, RG A-1, Corres., 1916, Box 14; Editorial, *Calif. St. Jour. Med.* 14 (Oct. 1916): 390–91; Rubinow, Remarks, ibid. 14 (Nov. 1916): 443. See also "Social Insurance," ibid. 14 (July 1916): 302–3, and open letter, René Bine to members of the state medical society, ibid. 14 (Aug. 1916): 306.

41. James L. Whitney, "Cooperative Medicine in Relation to Social Insurance, *Calif. St. Jour. Med.* 14 (Nov. 1916): 433, quotation, p. 434. Arthur J. Viseltear has traced the origins of Whitney's paper to earlier articles by Michael M. Davis, Jr., and Alexander Lambert (see "Compulsory Health Insurance in California, 1915–18," *Jour. Hist. Med.* 24 [April 1969]: 161n). For another instance of a California physician citing the limitations of the fee-for-service system and charging that "the average working man is too poorly paid to properly compensate a doctor for his time and trouble through serious illness," see Morton Raymond Gibbons, "Social Insurance," *Calif. St. Jour. Med.* 15 (Feb. 1917): 48. This paper was read before the Los Angeles County Medical Society, 9 Nov. 1916. Gibbons favored a compulsory system if it contained certain safeguards protecting physicians and patients.

42. Frank Billings and C. D. Selby, Remarks, *Amer. Labor. Leg. Rev.* 7 (March 1917): 54, 55; *JAMA* 99 (1 Oct. 1932): 1187.

43. Frederick R. Green, Remarks, *Amer. Labor Leg. Rev.* 7 (March 1917): 56.

44. Alexander Lambert, "Medical Organization under Health Insurance," *Amer. Labor. Leg. Rev.* 7 (March 1917): 37, 46–48; Irving Fisher, "The Need for Health Insurance," ibid., p. 11; Form letter, Andrews to "Dear Doctor," 21 Dec. 1916, Andrews Papers RG A-1, Corres., 1916, Box 15; "Medical Service in Health Insurance," *JAMA* 67 (30 Dec. 1916): 2032.

45. *Amer. Labor Leg. Rev.* 7 (March 1917): 207; *Report of Special Commission on Insurance* [Massachusetts], Feb. 1917, House No. 1850 (Boston, 1917), pp. 7–8, quotation, p. 16.

46. *Report on Health Insurance by the New Jersey Commission on Old Age, Insurance and Pensions*, p. 1; State of Connecticut, *Report of the Commission on Public Welfare* (Hartford, 1919), p. 3; Borah to Andrews, 22 Jan. 1917, Andrews Papers, RG A-1, Corres., 1917–18, Box 16; *Amer. Labor Leg. Rev.* 7 (March 1917): 208, 224, 225; *Calif. St. Med. Jour.* 16 (July 1918): 348. Hiram Johnson, who had served as governor of California since January 1911, was elected to the United States Senate in November 1916 for the session beginning in March 1917. He pre-

ferred to remain as governor until 15 March and was succeeded by the lieutenant governor, William D. Stephens. While Johnson recommended compulsory health insurance in his legislative address, 8 January 1917, insurance proponents detected that some of his enthusiasm for the proposal had waned (Viseltear, "Compulsory Health Insurance," pp. 168–69).

47. "Compulsory Health Insurance," *JAMA* 68 (27 Jan. 1917): 292; Alexander Lambert, "Health Insurance and the Medical Profession," ibid., p. 257.

48. Irving Fisher, "The Need for Health Insurance," *N.Y. St. Jour. Med.* 17 (Feb. 1917): 80–84; undated three-page manuscript, Rubinow Papers, RG A-3, Corres., PI-RZ, Box 7.

49. *New York Times Magazine,* 30 Jan. 1916, p. 8; I. M. Rubinow, *Health Insurance in Relation to the Public Dispensary,* Social Insurance Series, Pamphlet No. 3 (Chicago: American Medical Association), pp. 3, 5; Delphey to Andrews, 26 Feb. 1916, Andrews Papers, RG A-1, Corres., 1916, Box 14; "Opposition to the Health Insurance Bill," (Editorial), *Med. Record* 89 (4 March 1916): 423. The editor of the *Medical Record* strongly protested the hasty action of the Medical Society of the County of New York in denouncing the bill, declaring that "blind condemnation will lead nowhere" (ibid., p. 424).

50. OSH to Rooney, 23 March 1916; Andrews to Rooney, 24 March 1916, Andrews Papers RG A-1, Corres., 1916, Box 14; quotations, "Report of the Chairman of the Committee on Legislation of the Medical Society of the County of New York," *N.Y. St. Jour. Med.* 16 (March 1916): 157, 158, and OSH to Lambert, 16 March 1916, Andrews Papers, RG A-1, Corres., 1916, Box 14; Andrews to Joseph P. Chamberlain, 31 March 1916, and Minutes of Social Insurance Committee of AALL, 22 April 1916, Andrews Papers, RG A-1, Corres., 1916, Box 14. For accounts of conferences between spokesmen for the AALL and the two New York societies see two three-page reports in Andrews Papers, RG A-1, Corres., 1916, Box 15.

51. The Massachusetts commission had been created before early June 1916, and the *New York Times* observed, "It is an open secret that if health insurance becomes obligatory in New York, Massachusetts may follow, and that every effort will be made to incorporate it among the statutes of each state of the Union, thus making its application national in every sense" (*New York Times Magazine,* 30 Jan. 1916, p. 8). See also OSH to Herbert Croly, 10 June 1916, Andrews Papers, RG A-1, Corres., 1916, Box 15.

52. E. R. Hayhurst to Andrews, 27 May 1916, Andrews Papers, RG A-1, Corres., 1916, Box 14; Grant Hamilton, "Proposed Legislation for Health Insurance," Department of Labor, *Proceedings of the Conference on Social Insurance,* 1916, p. 564; Edson S. Lott, "Fallacies of Compulsory Social Insurance," *Western Review* 23 (April 1917): 4.

53. Editorial, *JAMA* 73 (2 Dec. 1916): 1677; Jones to Andrews, 22 April 1916 and 26 May 1916, Andrews Papers, RG A-1, Corres., 1916, Box. 14.

54. Andrews to Hoffman, 19 Dec. 1916, p. 6, Andrews Papers, RG A-1, Corres., 1916, Box 15. This letter acknowledged receipt of Hoffman's letter of 11 December, confirming his resignation a few days earlier. Hoffman apparently submitted a resignation in early 1916 but for some reason retained an official connection with the AALL until December (see Irving Fisher to Andrews, 13 April 1916, Andrews Papers, RG A-1, Corres., 1916). Fisher wrote very frankly to Hoffman calling into question the latter's assertion that his connection with a major life insurance company had not affected his attitude toward health insurance. Fisher said that an undisclosed mutual friend had told him, "Of coure you can't believe that, however hard you try" (Fisher to Hoffman, 9 Feb. 1917, Andrews Papers, RG A-1, Corres., 1916–17,

Box 16). At the social insurance conference earlier in the year Hoffman said that he had already closed his connection with the AALL (see Department of Labor, *Proceedings of the Conference on Social Insurance*, 1916, p. 624).

55. Commons, "Health Insurance," p. 222.

56. Department of Labor, *Proceedings of the Conference on Social Insurance,* 1916, p. 624.

57. Frederick L. Hoffman, *Facts and Fallacies of Compulsory Health Insurance* (Newark: Prudential Press, 1917), p. 5.

58. Donald M. Gedge, "The Proposed Social Health Insurance Act," *Calif. St. Jour. Med.* 14 (Nov. 1916): 446, 447, for the two quotations.

59. Quotations, Hoffman, "Some Fallacies of Health Insurance," Press Release, 23 Jan. 1917, by the National Civic Federation, Andrews Papers, RG A-1 Health Insurance, Box 70; Frederick L. Hoffman, "Public Health Progress under Social Insurance," *Insurance and Commercial Magazine* 82 (Feb. 1917): 28.

60. William Gale Curtis, *Social Insurance,* Bulletin No. 5 (Insurance Economic Society of America), p. 4, Andrews Papers, RG A-1, Health Insurance, Box 70.

61. *Who's Who in America,* vol. 7 (1912–13), p. 1899; quotations, *Criticism of a Tentative Draft of an Act for Health Insurance* (New York, 1917), p. 10.

62. Hoffman, *Facts and Fallacies,* pp. 13–14. The Legislative Committee of the National Civic Federation in *Compulsory Health Insurance,* a twenty-two page pamphlet, raised sixteen objections to the Mills bill (Andrews Papers, RG A-1, Health Insurance, Box 70). A physician, Henry W. Berg, representing the Real Estate Owners' Association of New York City, said at hearings before the Senate Judiciary Committee, "The backers of the bill got it straight from Germany and you know to what such paternalism has led all over Europe" (*New York Times,* 5 March 1917, p. 7). For an account of opposition of insurance companies in the city of New York see Isaac M. Rubinow, letter to the editor, *JAMA* 68 (28 April 1917): 1279.

63. Frederick L. Hoffman, "Compulsory Health Insurance Unnecessary as a Public Health Measure," *JAMA* 68 (10 Feb. 1917): 480; "Objections to Social or Compulsory Health Insurance by the Committee on Health Insurance," *Ill. Med. Jour.* 31 (March 1917): 188–94. The AMA's House of Delegates at its annual session in June 1917 accepted four specific requirements for any health insurance plan that the AMA's Subcommittee on Social Insurance had drafted. These included free choice of physicians, their payment in proportion to the amount of work they performed, separation of medical supervisory functions from the daily care of the sick, and adequate representation of the profession in the administration of the law ("Report of Committee on Social Insurance," *JAMA* 68 [9 June 1917]: 1755; ibid. 68 [16 June 1917]: 1852).

64. "Report of Committee on Compulsory Health Insurance," *Calif. St. Jour. Med.* 15 (June 1917): 194–98; quotation, "Report of Committee on New Business," ibid., p. 22, adopted, p. 199.

65. Many years later Rubinow said that inclusion of funeral benefits in the model bill accounted for much of the opposition of insurance companies. See Isaac M. Rubinow, "Do We Need Compulsory Public Health Insurance?" *Annals of the American Academy of Political and Social Science* 170 (Nov. 1933): 116. For details of the abortive postwar crusade see Odin W. Anderson, "Health Insurance in the United States, 1910–1920," *Jour. Hist. Med.* 5 (Autumn 1950): 378–94.

66. See Chapter 8 for details of the struggle against contract practice.

67. George MacAdams, "Do We Want to Pay the Health Insurance Bill?" *New York Times Magazine,* 11 March 1917, p. 11.

INDEX

American Society of Medical Economics, 130, 141
Andrews, John B., 139, 141, 143, 147, 149
Arena, 3
Arizona, 7, 63, 90
Arkansas, 43, 56, 61
Arndt, Hugo R., 79–80
Association of American Medical Colleges, 35, 67

Barker, N. L., 109
Baton Rouge, La., 100
Bay City, Mich., 121
Beates, Henry, Jr., 31
Beebe, Henry E., 74
Behring, Emil von, 8
Benedict, Arthur L., 124
Benevolent and fraternal orders, 120–23, 124–25, 126–28
Best, William P., 87
Bevan, Arthur D., 36, 44, 49
Bignami, Amigo, 5
Billings, Frank, 8, 93, 147
Billroch, Theodor, 40
Bixel, Peter D., 84
Blood research, 8, 10
Blumer, George, 145
Boards of health, 36, 44, 45, 59, 89, 90–91, 162
Bok, Edward, 115
Boston: dispensaries, 112; healing groups, 53–54; school medical inspection, 93
Borah, William E., 148
Bowling Green, Ky., 115
Boyle, Emmet W., 148
Brewer, David J., 67
Brigham, Peter Bent, 12
British National Health Insurance System, 140, 143
Brooks, John Graham, 133
Brotherhood of St. John, 121
Brown, Rexwald, 127
Bubonic plague, 5, 8
Buffalo, N.Y.: cancer laboratory, 98; fraternal orders, 120
Durnham, Athel C., 145
Butler, Pa., 7

California: contract practice, 125, 127–28; eclectic medicine, 82, 86; epidemics, 5, 7; fraternal orders, 121–22; health insurance, 146, 147; licensure, 59; medical examiners, 31, 61; medical practice act, 64; medical society, 5, 96, 125; milk inspection, 96; sterilization, 99; and Supreme Court, 67; and workmen's compensation, 135, 136
California State Journal of Medicine, 122, 131, 135, 142, 146, 150
Canada, 40
Cancer: and Christian Science, 57; and mortality, 7, 90; research, 9, 97–98
Capper, Arthur, 69
Carbondale, Pa., 109
Cardiology, 9
Carlisle Co. (Kentucky) Medical Society, 110, 164–65
Carnegie, Andrew, 11, 46
Carnegie Foundation for the Advancement of Teaching, 12, 42, 44, 47–48, 66, 78
Carnegie Institute, 11
Casualty, Actuarial and Statistical Society of America, 146
Census Bureau, 100
Chamberlain, Joseph P., 141
Charity patients, 24, 111–13, 163
Chicago: AMA conference, 33–34; contract practice, 122, 123; dispensaries, 111–12; medical schools, 43; medical society, 112; public school inspection, 93
Children's Bureau, 101
Chiropractors, 53, 55–56; licensure of, 59, 60; and medical practice acts, 64, 69–70; and schools, 57
Cholera, 24
Christian Science, 53–54; and licensure, 59, 60–61; and national health department, 101
Churchill, John E., 46
Cincinnati: eclectic medicine, 82–83, 85, 87; milk inspection, 95–96; school inspection, 94–95
Cities: contract practice, 120–22; and diseases, 5, 7; and dispensaries, 111–13; and milk inspection, 95–96; and school inspection, 93, 94–95
Clary, Lloyd A., 114

THE JOHNS HOPKINS UNIVERSITY PRESS

This book was composed in Linotype Caledonia text and
Century Expanded Bold display type by Keith Press, Inc., from
a design by Susan Bishop. It was printed and bound by The
Murray Printing Company.

LIBRARY OF CONGRESS CATALOGING IN PUBLICATION DATA

Burrow, James Gordon, 1922–
    Organized medicine in the progressive era.

    Bibliography: pp. 168–69
    Includes index.
    1. Medicine—United States—History.   2. Medical societies—United States—
Political activity—History.   3. Medical economics—United States—History.
4. Progressivism (United States politics)   I. Title. DNLM: 1. History of
medicine, 20th century—U. S.   2. Politics.   WZ70 AA1 B90

R152.B8   362.1'0973   77–894
ISBN 0–8018–1918–0